The Hormone Reset Plan: Balance Your Body, Reclaim Your Energy, Transform Your Life

A Unique 4-Week Blueprint to Revitalize Your Thyroid, Adrenals, Mood, and Metabolism Naturally

Nelson Andrew

Table of Contents

Chapter 1: Understanding Hormonal Imbalance
1.1 What Are Hormones and Why They Matter
1.2 Signs and Symptoms of Hormonal Imbalance
1.3 The Hidden Causes: Stress, Diet, and Environment

Chapter 2: The Hormone Reset Blueprint
2.1 How the 4-Week Plan Works
2.2 Preparing for Success: Setting Goals and Clearing Your Space
2.3 Tracking Your Progress: Key Metrics to Monitor

Week 1: Cleanse and Nourish

Chapter 3: Eliminating Hormonal Disruptors
3.1 Foods That Hurt: What to Avoid

3.2 Cleaning Up Your Environment: Toxins to Eliminate
3.3 The Daily Detox Ritual: Simple Cleansing Practices

Chapter 4: Fueling Your Body with Nutrients
4.1 The Power of Anti-Inflammatory Foods
4.2 Building Your Plate: A Practical Meal Guide
4.3 Hormone-Boosting Smoothies and Beverages

Week 2: Rebuild and Stabilize

Chapter 5: Stabilizing Blood Sugar and Insulin
5.1 The Blood Sugar-Hormone Connection
5.2 Balanced Meals: Combining Protein, Fat, and Fiber
5.3 Snack Smart: Easy, Hormone-Friendly Snacks

Chapter 6: Gentle Movement and Stress Relief
6.1 Exercises That Balance Hormones

6.2 The Art of Stress Management: Mindfulness and Relaxation
6.3 Restoring Energy with Adaptogens

Week 3: Restore and Recharge

Chapter 7: Supporting Thyroid and Adrenal Health
7.1 Foods and Nutrients for Thyroid Support
7.2 Replenishing Adrenal Reserves Naturally
7.3 Supplements for Energy and Balance

Chapter 8: Building Restful Sleep and Recovery
8.1 The Sleep-Hormone Connection
8.2 Creating a Bedtime Routine That Heals

Week 4: Sustain and Thrive

Chapter 9: Maintaining Hormonal Balance Long-Term
9.1 Reinforcing Healthy Habits
9.2 Adapting to Seasonal and Life Changes
9.3 Setting Up a Weekly Self-Care Routine

Chapter 10: Detoxifying Your Lifestyle
10.1 Transitioning to Clean Personal Care Products
10.2 DIY Natural Cleaning Solutions
10.3 Reducing Environmental Stressors

Chapter 1

Understanding Hormonal Imbalance

1.1 What Are Hormones and Why They Matter

Hormones are chemical messengers produced by glands in the endocrine system, and they play a critical role in regulating nearly every function in your body. Though you cannot see or feel them directly, these tiny, powerful substances influence how you grow, feel, sleep, eat, and even think. Hormones are essential for maintaining balance in the body, ensuring that all its systems work harmoniously together.

The Basics of Hormones

Hormones are secreted directly into the bloodstream by glands such as the thyroid, adrenal glands, pancreas, ovaries, and testes. Once released, they travel to specific organs and tissues to deliver instructions. Each hormone has a unique job, and even small fluctuations in hormone levels can have significant effects on your body and mind.

For example:

- Insulin, produced by the pancreas, regulates blood sugar levels.

- Estrogen and testosterone, produced in the ovaries and testes respectively, control sexual and reproductive health.

- Thyroid hormones influence metabolism, energy levels, and body temperature.

- Cortisol, the stress hormone, helps your body respond to challenges but can cause problems when chronically elevated.

Why Hormones Matter

Hormones are integral to your overall health and well-being. **They control key processes such as:**

1. Growth and Development
From infancy to adulthood, hormones like growth hormone guide physical development, helping bones, muscles, and tissues grow properly.

2. Metabolism and Energy Regulation
Hormones ensure your body converts food into energy efficiently. Imbalances can lead to issues like weight gain, fatigue, or conditions such as diabetes.

3. Reproductive Health
Hormones regulate menstrual cycles, fertility, pregnancy, and even libido. They are crucial for the continuation of life and maintaining sexual health.

4. Mood and Mental Health

Hormones like serotonin and dopamine affect your emotions, while cortisol and adrenaline influence your stress responses. Imbalances can contribute to anxiety, depression, or mood swings.

5. Sleep and Recovery

Melatonin, the sleep hormone, governs your sleep-wake cycle, ensuring you get restorative rest. Growth hormone also supports tissue repair during sleep.

6. Immune Function

Hormones like cortisol have a hand in your immune response, determining how your body fights infections or heals injuries.

The Impact of Hormonal Imbalances

When hormones are out of balance, the effects can ripple through every system in your body. **Common signs of hormonal imbalances include:**

- Unexplained weight gain or loss

- Fatigue or low energy levels

- Mood swings, anxiety, or depression

- Difficulty sleeping

- Irregular menstrual cycles or infertility

- Skin issues, like acne or dryness

Left untreated, these imbalances can lead to chronic health conditions such as polycystic ovary syndrome (PCOS), thyroid disorders, or metabolic syndrome.

Supporting Healthy Hormones

Maintaining hormonal balance requires a combination of healthy lifestyle choices:

1. Nutrition: A balanced diet with whole foods, healthy fats, and limited sugar supports hormone production.

2. Exercise: Regular physical activity helps regulate insulin, cortisol, and other key hormones.

3. Stress Management: Chronic stress disrupts hormone levels, so practices like mindfulness, yoga, or deep breathing can help.

4. Sleep: Quality sleep is critical for hormonal health. Aim for 7-9 hours per night.

5. Avoid Toxins: Reduce exposure to environmental toxins found in plastics, processed foods, and certain skincare products, as they can disrupt hormones.

Hormones are the foundation of your body's internal communication system, influencing nearly every aspect of your health. Understanding how they work and taking steps to support their balance is essential for achieving optimal physical, emotional, and mental well-being. By prioritizing a healthy lifestyle, you can help your hormones work harmoniously, allowing you to thrive.

1.2 Signs and Symptoms of Hormonal Imbalance

Hormones are chemical messengers that regulate nearly every function in the body, from energy levels and metabolism to mood and reproductive health. When hormones are out of balance, even slightly, it can create a ripple effect, leading to a range of noticeable symptoms. **Below is a clear and comprehensive look at the signs and symptoms of hormonal imbalance.**

1. Unexplained Weight Changes

Weight Gain: Hormonal imbalances, particularly in cortisol (stress hormone) or insulin, can make it difficult to manage weight. Thyroid issues, like hypothyroidism, can also slow metabolism, leading to weight gain.

Weight Loss: On the flip side, an overactive thyroid (hyperthyroidism) can cause unexplained weight loss despite eating normally.

2. Fatigue and Low Energy

Feeling constantly tired, even after a full night's sleep, could indicate a hormonal issue. Cortisol imbalances caused by stress or thyroid dysfunction may result in persistent fatigue.

3. Mood Swings and Irritability

Hormones like estrogen, progesterone, and testosterone influence brain chemistry. Imbalances can lead to mood swings, irritability, anxiety, or even depression. Women experiencing menopause or PMS often notice these emotional changes due to fluctuating hormone levels.

4. Sleep Problems

Insomnia: Low progesterone or elevated cortisol can disrupt sleep patterns, making it hard to fall or stay asleep.

Oversleeping: Conversely, hypothyroidism may lead to excessive sleepiness or difficulty staying awake during the day.

5. Changes in Skin and Hair

Acne: Persistent adult acne, particularly along the jawline, is often linked to androgen (male hormone) imbalances, such as those seen in polycystic ovary syndrome (PCOS).

Hair Loss: Thinning hair or bald spots can result from imbalances in thyroid hormones, testosterone, or estrogen.

Dry Skin: Low thyroid function can cause skin to become dry, flaky, and prone to irritation.

6. Irregular or Painful Menstrual Cycles

For women, hormonal imbalance often affects the menstrual cycle:

•Skipped, irregular, or heavy periods may signal problems with estrogen or progesterone.

•Severe cramping, bloating, or PMS symptoms can indicate imbalances in reproductive hormones.

7. Low Libido or Sexual Dysfunction

A decline in testosterone in men and women can result in reduced sexual desire. Hormonal imbalances can also lead to issues like erectile dysfunction in men or vaginal dryness in women.

8. Digestive Issues

Hormones regulate digestion, so imbalances may cause bloating, diarrhea, or constipation. Stress-related cortisol surges, for instance, often affect gut health.

9. Increased Sensitivity to Temperature

People with thyroid hormone imbalances may feel unusually cold (hypothyroidism) or hot (hyperthyroidism), even in normal temperatures.

10. Appetite and Cravings

Hormones like leptin and ghrelin control hunger. Imbalances can lead to intense cravings or an inability to feel full, contributing to overeating or poor food choices.

11. Chronic Stress or Anxiety

Cortisol dysregulation due to ongoing stress can lead to feelings of being constantly overwhelmed, anxious, or unable to relax.

12. Changes in Breasts

In women, hormonal fluctuations can cause breast tenderness, lumpiness, or swelling.

Persistent changes may signal hormonal conditions that require medical attention.

13. Infertility or Difficulty Conceiving

Hormonal imbalances are a common cause of infertility in both men and women. Issues like PCOS, low testosterone, or thyroid dysfunction can disrupt ovulation or sperm production.

14. Weakened Bones

Hormones like estrogen and testosterone play a vital role in bone density. Imbalances, particularly after menopause, can lead to brittle or weak bones (osteoporosis).

15. Brain Fog and Memory Problems

Hormonal imbalances can affect cognitive function, causing forgetfulness, difficulty concentrating, or a "foggy" feeling. This is especially common with thyroid or menopause-related hormonal shifts.

The signs and symptoms of hormonal imbalance vary widely and can affect multiple areas of health. While occasional imbalances are normal, persistent or severe symptoms should not be ignored. Consulting a healthcare provider is essential for proper diagnosis and treatment. Balancing hormones often requires a holistic approach, including lifestyle changes, proper nutrition, stress management, and, in some cases, medical intervention.

Recognizing the symptoms is the first step to reclaiming your health and well-being.

1.3 The Hidden Causes: Stress, Diet, and Environment

Hormones regulate critical functions in the body, from metabolism and sleep to mood and reproduction. When these chemical messengers fall out of sync, the effects can be life-disrupting. To tackle this problem effectively, it's essential to understand the often-overlooked root causes: **stress, diet, and environmental factors.**

1. The Role of Stress in Hormonal Imbalance

Chronic stress is one of the most significant yet underestimated contributors to hormonal imbalance. When the body perceives stress—whether from work pressure, relationship problems, or financial challenges—it activates the "fight or flight" response. This leads to the release of cortisol, a stress hormone produced by the adrenal glands.

While short bursts of cortisol are essential for survival, prolonged stress keeps cortisol levels elevated, which disrupts other hormonal systems. **For example:**

Thyroid Function: Chronic stress can suppress thyroid hormones, leading to fatigue, weight gain, and depression.

Reproductive Health: High cortisol levels interfere with sex hormones like estrogen, progesterone, and testosterone, causing irregular periods, low libido, and fertility issues.

Blood Sugar Regulation: Elevated cortisol prompts the liver to release more glucose, increasing the risk of insulin resistance and weight gain.

Reducing stress is vital. Practices like mindfulness meditation, deep breathing exercises, regular physical activity, and prioritizing rest can help restore balance.

2. Diet: The Foundation of Hormonal Health

Your diet directly influences hormone production, regulation, and overall health. Modern dietary habits, often high in processed foods, sugar, and unhealthy fats, wreak havoc on the endocrine system. **Here's how diet affects hormones:**

Excess Sugar and Refined Carbs: A diet rich in sugary snacks and white flour spikes insulin levels. Over time, this can lead to insulin resistance, a precursor to diabetes and a disruptor of sex hormones.

Inflammatory Foods: Trans fats, processed meats, and artificial additives trigger inflammation, which interferes with hormone signaling.

Nutrient Deficiencies: Hormone production requires essential nutrients like zinc, magnesium, and vitamins B, D, and E. A diet lacking in these can lead to imbalances.

Gut Health: The gut microbiome plays a pivotal role in hormone metabolism. An unhealthy gut, often caused by poor diet or overuse of antibiotics, can lead to improper hormone regulation, particularly of estrogen.

To support hormonal health, focus on:

Whole Foods: Fresh fruits, vegetables, whole grains, and lean proteins.

Healthy Fats: Avocado, nuts, seeds, and fatty fish, which aid in hormone production.

Balanced Meals: Combine protein, healthy fats, and fiber at every meal to stabilize blood sugar and reduce insulin spikes.

Hydration: Water supports detoxification, helping the body eliminate excess hormones and toxins.

3. Environmental Toxins: The Silent Saboteurs

Our environment is filled with chemicals and pollutants that mimic hormones or disrupt the body's hormonal systems. These substances, known as endocrine disruptors, are found in everyday products like plastics, cosmetics, cleaning supplies, and even food packaging.

Plastics and BPA: Bisphenol A (BPA) and similar chemicals in plastic containers and water bottles act like estrogen in the body, leading to hormone imbalance and even fertility issues.

Pesticides and Herbicides: Many chemicals used in agriculture disrupt thyroid function and reproductive hormones.

Personal Care Products: Phthalates, parabens, and synthetic fragrances in cosmetics and shampoos mimic or interfere with hormone production.

Household Cleaners: Toxic fumes and harsh chemicals burden the liver, which plays a key role in hormone detoxification.

To reduce exposure:

•Use glass or stainless-steel containers instead of plastic.

•Choose organic produce whenever possible to minimize pesticide exposure.

•Switch to natural, fragrance-free personal care and cleaning products.

•Ensure proper ventilation in your home to reduce indoor air pollution.

The Path to Balance

Addressing stress, improving diet, and minimizing environmental toxins are powerful steps to restoring hormonal balance. While it's tempting to look for quick fixes, the most lasting solutions come from lifestyle changes.

Start small. Swap processed foods for whole, nutrient-rich options. Dedicate a few minutes daily to stress-reducing activities. Replace chemical-laden products with natural alternatives. Over time, these small shifts create a ripple effect that transforms your health.

Remember, hormonal imbalance is not a life sentence. By understanding and addressing the hidden causes, you can regain control of your body, improve your well-being, and live with vitality and balance.

Chapter 2

The Hormone Reset Blueprint

2.1 How the 4-Week Plan Works

This plan is designed to reset your hormones and rejuvenate your energy levels through a structured, natural, and holistic approach. By breaking down the journey into manageable weekly goals, it simplifies the process of balancing your hormones while addressing the root causes of common imbalances. Each week builds upon the last, targeting specific aspects of hormonal health for lasting change. **Here's a comprehensive overview of how the 4-week plan works.**

Week 1: Cleanse and Nourish

The first week is all about cleansing your body of toxins and replenishing it with nourishing foods and habits. By eliminating hormonal disruptors and introducing detoxifying practices, you'll lay the foundation for hormonal balance.

Week 2: Rebuild and Stabilize

After cleansing, the second week focuses on rebuilding your hormonal foundation and stabilizing blood sugar levels, which are key to hormonal harmony.

Week 3: Restore and Recharge

This week focuses on restoring the health of your thyroid and adrenal glands while improving sleep quality to recharge your body.

Week 4: Sustain and Thrive

In the final week, you'll focus on maintaining the habits you've built and creating a sustainable lifestyle for long-term hormonal health.

This four-week plan provides a clear and actionable roadmap to balance your hormones and reclaim your vitality. By making small, intentional changes each week, you'll create a lasting foundation for health, energy, and well-being.

2.2 Preparing for Success: Setting Goals and Clearing Your Space

Before embarking on the 4-week hormone reset plan, it's essential to prepare your mind, body, and environment for success. A strong foundation ensures you stay focused, motivated, and equipped to follow through with the plan. By setting clear goals and creating a supportive space, you'll increase your chances of achieving lasting results.

Setting Goals for Your Hormone Reset Journey

1. Define Your "Why"

Start by asking yourself why you want to reset your hormones. Are you seeking more energy, better sleep, improved mood, or weight balance? Identifying your primary motivation will keep you grounded and determined when challenges arise. Write down your "why" and keep it visible as a daily reminder.

2. Set Clear, Measurable Goals
Create specific, achievable goals for the next four weeks. **For example:**

✓ "I will prepare three hormone-friendly meals per day."

✓ "I will practice mindfulness or yoga for 10 minutes daily."

✓ "I will avoid processed foods and sugary snacks."

Break larger goals into smaller, actionable steps. Instead of aiming to eliminate all toxins at once, start by replacing one or two products each week.

3. Track Your Progress

Use a journal, planner, or app to record daily habits, meals, energy levels, and any noticeable changes. Reflecting on your progress helps you stay accountable and adapt as needed.

Clearing Your Space for Success

Your physical environment plays a critical role in your ability to succeed. A clutter-free, toxin-free space reduces stress, supports your goals, and creates an atmosphere of renewal.

1. Detox Your Kitchen
Go through your pantry and refrigerator to remove items that don't align with the plan. **These include:**

✓ Processed snacks

✓ Sugary beverages

✓ Refined oils and flours

✓ Foods with artificial additives or preservatives

Stock your kitchen with fresh vegetables, fruits, whole grains, lean proteins, healthy fats, and hormone-boosting spices like turmeric and cinnamon. Organize your shelves and storage spaces to make healthy choices easily accessible.

2. Simplify Your Living Space
A cluttered environment can lead to feelings of overwhelm and stress, which may negatively impact your hormone health. **Dedicate a weekend to decluttering your home:**

✓ Remove items that no longer serve you.

✓ Organize essentials into neat, easy-to-access spaces.

✓ Introduce calming elements like plants, soft lighting, and soothing scents.

3. Replace Toxic Products
Eliminate products containing hormone-disrupting chemicals, such as parabens,

phthalates, and synthetic fragrances. **Start with these categories:**

Personal Care: Switch to clean shampoos, soaps, and moisturizers.

Cleaning Products: Replace chemical-heavy cleaners with DIY natural solutions like vinegar and baking soda.

Plastics: Use glass or stainless steel for food storage and water bottles to avoid BPA and phthalates.

4. Create a Relaxation Zone
Designate a corner or room in your home for relaxation and mindfulness practices. Add a yoga mat, cozy blanket, journal, or meditation cushion. This space will serve as your sanctuary for stress relief and hormone-friendly activities.

Mindset Matters: Visualizing Your Success

As you prepare, spend time visualizing the results you hope to achieve. Imagine yourself feeling energized, balanced, and confident. Use affirmations to reinforce positive changes.

Preparing for success is the first step toward achieving hormonal balance and reclaiming your energy. By setting clear goals, clearing your space, and fostering a positive mindset, you'll be ready to fully embrace the 4-week plan and transform your life naturally.

2.3 Tracking Your Progress: Key Metrics to Monitor

Tracking your progress is an essential part of the 4-week hormone reset plan. It not only helps you stay accountable but also provides insights into the effectiveness of the changes you're making. By observing specific metrics, you can identify patterns, make adjustments, and celebrate small wins along the way. This section outlines the key areas to monitor and offers practical tips for keeping track of your progress.

1. Energy Levels

Hormonal imbalances often cause fatigue and low energy. As you implement the plan, pay attention to changes in how energized you feel throughout the day.

How to Monitor:

Keep a daily energy log. Rate your energy levels on a scale of 1 to 10 at morning, midday, and evening.

Note any patterns, such as consistent afternoon crashes, and correlate them with meals, stress levels, or sleep quality.

Reflect weekly to identify improvements or areas needing adjustment.

What to Look For:

✓ Increased morning energy.

✓ Fewer dips in energy throughout the day.

✓ Sustained stamina during physical activities.

2. Mood and Emotional Well-Being

Hormones play a significant role in regulating mood. As your body begins to rebalance, you should notice fewer mood swings, less irritability, and an overall sense of calm.

How to Monitor:

Journal your feelings each day. Include notes on your stress levels, anxiety, or any sense of emotional stability.

Track how often you experience mood swings or intense emotional reactions.

Rate your overall mood on a scale of 1 to 10 at the end of each day.

What to Look For:

✓ A more positive, stable mood.

✓ Reduced stress and anxiety.

✓ Greater patience and emotional resilience.

3. Sleep Quality

Poor sleep disrupts hormone production, including cortisol, melatonin, and growth hormone. Restful, restorative sleep is a cornerstone of this plan.

How to Monitor:

Keep a sleep journal, **noting:**

The time you go to bed and wake up.

How many times you wake during the night.

How rested you feel upon waking.

Consider using a sleep tracker or app to measure sleep duration and quality.

What to Look For:

✓ Falling asleep faster and staying asleep longer.

✓ Waking up refreshed instead of groggy.

✓ Fewer disruptions in your sleep cycle.

4. Digestion and Gut Health

Your gut health directly impacts hormone regulation. Improved digestion is often an early sign that your body is responding well to dietary changes.

How to Monitor:

Keep a food and digestion diary. Note what you eat, how you feel after meals, and any symptoms like bloating, gas, or discomfort.

Track bowel movements using frequency, regularity, and ease as metrics.

What to Look For:

✓ Regular, comfortable digestion.

✓ Reduced bloating or stomach upset.

✓ Increased tolerance to nutrient-rich, hormone-supporting foods.

5. Weight and Body Composition

If weight management is part of your goal, observing gradual, sustainable changes in weight or body composition can reflect progress.

How to Monitor:

Weigh yourself no more than once a week to avoid becoming overly focused on numbers.

Track measurements of key areas like waist, hips, and chest.

Pay attention to how your clothes fit and your overall body tone.

What to Look For:

✓ Gradual weight loss (if applicable).

✓ Reduced water retention or bloating.

✓ Increased muscle tone and strength.

6. Skin Health

Hormones influence skin health, affecting conditions like acne, dryness, or oiliness. As you detoxify and nourish your body, your skin will often reflect the positive changes.

How to Monitor:

Take weekly photos of your skin in consistent lighting to track visible improvements.

Note changes in texture, clarity, and hydration in a skincare journal.

Record any reduction in symptoms like breakouts or redness.

What to Look For:

✓ Clearer, more radiant skin.

✓ Reduced inflammation or blemishes.

✓ Improved elasticity and hydration.

7. Menstrual Cycle or Hormonal Symptoms

For women, the menstrual cycle provides valuable insight into hormonal health. Improvements in cycle regularity and reduction in PMS symptoms indicate progress.

How to Monitor:

Track your cycle using an app or journal, noting start and end dates, flow heaviness, and symptoms like cramps or mood swings.

Monitor any changes in hormonal symptoms, such as breast tenderness, bloating, or fatigue.

What to Look For:

✓ More regular cycles.

✓ Lighter, less painful periods.

✓ Reduced PMS symptoms.

8. Overall Health and Well-Being

Beyond specific metrics, consider your overall sense of vitality and happiness. Hormonal balance often leads to subtle yet profound shifts in how you feel day-to-day.

How to Monitor:

Reflect on your general well-being each week in a journal.

Ask yourself: Do I feel stronger, calmer, or more focused than before?

Note any improvements in areas like mental clarity, resilience, or motivation.

What to Look For:

✓ A renewed sense of vitality.

✓ Greater mental clarity and focus.

✓ A more optimistic outlook on life.

Tips for Tracking Progress Effectively

1. Be Consistent: Track your metrics daily or weekly for the most accurate picture of your progress.

2. Celebrate Small Wins: Acknowledge and reward yourself for milestones, no matter how small.

3. Be Patient: Hormonal balance takes time. Focus on gradual improvements rather than immediate results.

4. Adjust When Needed: If progress stalls, use your tracking data to identify areas for refinement, such as tweaking your diet, adjusting exercise routines, or adding relaxation techniques.

By monitoring these key metrics, you'll gain valuable insights into your hormone reset journey. Tracking not only keeps you accountable but also helps you appreciate how far you've come, empowering you to stay committed to the process and enjoy the transformation.

Week 1: Cleanse and Nourish

Chapter 3

Eliminating Hormonal Disruptors

3.1 Foods That Hurt: What to Avoid

When it comes to resetting your hormones and achieving balance, what you don't eat can be just as important as what you do. Certain foods disrupt your delicate hormonal system, leading to fatigue, weight gain, mood swings, and other health challenges. Identifying and avoiding these triggers is a critical step in reclaiming your energy and transforming your life.

Here's a breakdown of foods to avoid during your hormone reset, along with the reasons why:

1. Refined Sugars and Sweeteners

Refined sugar is one of the biggest culprits in hormonal disruption. It causes blood sugar spikes, leading to insulin resistance—a precursor to type 2 diabetes and hormonal imbalances.

High sugar intake can also increase cortisol, the stress hormone, putting extra strain on your adrenal glands.

What to avoid:

✓ Candy, pastries, and baked goods

✓ Sugary beverages like soda and energy drinks

✓ Artificial sweeteners (aspartame, sucralose)

Why it matters:
Over time, excess sugar can lead to inflammation and weight gain, both of which contribute to conditions like polycystic ovary syndrome (PCOS) and thyroid imbalances.

2. Highly Processed Foods

Processed foods are packed with preservatives, additives, and unhealthy fats that disrupt your body's natural rhythms. They're often loaded with trans fats, which can interfere with hormone production and lead to inflammation.

What to avoid:

✓ Frozen meals and packaged snacks

✓ Chips, crackers, and processed cheese spreads

✓ Instant noodles and fast food

Why it matters:
Processed foods often lack the nutrients your body needs for hormone production, making it harder for your thyroid, adrenal glands, and reproductive system to function properly.

3. Gluten

For many, gluten—a protein found in wheat, barley, and rye—can trigger inflammation and gut issues. A leaky gut can interfere with nutrient absorption, impairing your body's ability to produce and regulate hormones effectively.

What to avoid:

✓ Bread, pasta, and baked goods made with wheat

✓ Beer and malt beverages

✓ Many sauces and dressings with hidden gluten

Why it matters:
In those with gluten sensitivity or celiac disease, gluten can exacerbate autoimmune conditions like Hashimoto's thyroiditis, which directly impacts hormone balance.

4. Dairy

While dairy can be nutritious for some, it's a common hormone disruptor for others. Conventional dairy often contains traces of synthetic hormones used in farming, which can interfere with your body's natural hormonal balance.

What to avoid:

✓ Milk, cheese, and yogurt from **non-organic** sources

✓ Ice cream and cream-based sauces

✓ Flavored dairy products with added sugars

Why it matters:
Dairy can increase inflammation and stimulate insulin-like growth factor 1 (IGF-1), a hormone that may contribute to hormonal acne and other imbalances.

5. Caffeine and Alcohol

While a morning coffee or evening glass of wine might seem harmless, both caffeine and alcohol can negatively impact your hormones. Caffeine increases cortisol levels, which can disrupt your adrenal health, while alcohol impairs liver function, making it harder to detoxify excess hormones.

What to avoid:

✓ Multiple cups of coffee per day

✓ Energy drinks and pre-workout supplements

✓ Wine, beer, and spirits

Why it matters:
Overconsumption of caffeine and alcohol can contribute to sleep disturbances, stress, and imbalances in estrogen, progesterone, and cortisol.

6. Industrial Seed Oils

Oils like soybean, corn, and canola are often highly processed and rich in omega-6 fatty acids, which promote inflammation when consumed in excess. A diet high in these oils can disrupt the balance between omega-3 and omega-6 fatty acids, essential for hormone health.

What to avoid:

✓ Fried foods

✓ Packaged dressings and mayonnaise

✓ Foods cooked in vegetable oil

Why it matters:
A diet heavy in omega-6 oils can lead to chronic inflammation, impacting your thyroid and reproductive hormones.

7. Soy Products

Soy contains phytoestrogens, plant compounds that mimic estrogen in the body. While some soy can be beneficial in moderation, excessive consumption may disrupt hormonal balance, particularly in those with estrogen-dominant conditions.

What to avoid:

✓ Soy milk, soy protein isolate, and tofu (in large amounts)

✓ Processed soy products like soy burgers and soy-based snacks

✓ Soy sauces with high sodium

Why it matters:
Overconsumption of soy can interfere with thyroid function and exacerbate hormonal imbalances in sensitive individuals.

8. Foods with Artificial Additives

Artificial colors, flavors, and preservatives can overwhelm your liver, which plays a crucial role in metabolizing and detoxifying hormones. A burdened liver can lead to an accumulation of excess estrogen and other hormonal imbalances.

What to avoid:

✓ Packaged snacks with long ingredient lists

✓ Diet foods labeled "sugar-free" or "low-fat"

✓ Candies and sodas with bright artificial colors

Why it matters:
Reducing your intake of artificial ingredients supports liver health, which is essential for proper hormone regulation.

The Bottom Line

Eliminating these harmful foods during your hormone reset will allow your body to heal, rebalance, and thrive. Avoiding these disruptors isn't about restriction—it's about giving your body the best possible environment for transformation.

As you follow this plan, focus on replacing these foods with nutrient-dense, whole-food alternatives. Every positive choice you make brings you closer to revitalized energy, better health, and a thriving hormonal system.

Your journey to balance starts with what's on your plate—choose wisely, and your body will thank you.

3.2 Cleaning Up Your Environment: Toxins to Eliminate

Our everyday environments are filled with hidden toxins that can disrupt your hormones, sap your energy, and hinder your ability to feel and function at your best. Cleaning up your environment is a foundational step in balancing your body and restoring vitality. **Here's how to identify and eliminate the most common culprits to create a hormone-friendly home and lifestyle.**

1. Household Cleaners

Conventional cleaning products often contain harsh chemicals like phthalates, formaldehyde, and ammonia. These substances can interfere with hormone function, irritate the skin, and pollute indoor air.

Solution:

Replace toxic cleaners with natural alternatives such as vinegar, baking soda, and castile soap.

Look for eco-friendly, fragrance-free options labeled "non-toxic" or "biodegradable."

DIY recipes are also a great way to control what goes into your cleaning solutions.

2. Personal Care Products

Shampoos, lotions, makeup, and deodorants often contain endocrine disruptors like parabens, sulfates, and synthetic fragrances. These can mimic hormones in the body, leading to imbalances over time.

Solution:

Choose products made with organic, plant-based ingredients.

Avoid labels that list "fragrance" or "perfume" without clarification.

Use fewer products overall—simplifying your routine can minimize exposure.

3. Plastic Containers and Packaging

Plastics, particularly those containing BPA or phthalates, can leach hormone-disrupting chemicals into food, beverages, and the air. Even BPA-free plastics may still pose risks.

Solution:

Switch to glass, stainless steel, or silicone containers for food storage and water bottles.

Avoid microwaving food in plastic, as heat increases chemical leaching.

Minimize plastic use by buying fresh, unpackaged produce when possible.

4. Processed Foods

Processed and packaged foods are often loaded with preservatives, artificial colors, and chemical additives, which can overburden your body's detox systems and disrupt hormones. Additionally, the high levels of sugar and unhealthy fats can trigger inflammation and weight gain, further impacting hormonal health.

Solution:

Focus on whole, unprocessed foods like fresh fruits, vegetables, nuts, seeds, and lean proteins.

Read ingredient labels carefully—choose products with simple, recognizable components.

Limit sugar and processed snacks to reduce stress on your metabolism and thyroid.

5. Water Contaminants

Tap water can carry traces of heavy metals, pesticides, chlorine, and other chemicals that affect thyroid and adrenal function. These substances can also interfere with the body's detox pathways.

Solution:

Invest in a high-quality water filter that removes heavy metals, chlorine, and fluoride.

Use filtered water for both drinking and cooking.

Consider testing your home's water supply for specific toxins.

6. Air Pollutants

Indoor air pollution from synthetic fragrances, mold, dust, and volatile organic compounds

(VOCs) in paint and furniture can wreak havoc on your respiratory system and hormones.

Solution:

Ventilate your home daily by opening windows and using exhaust fans.

Add air-purifying plants like peace lilies or snake plants to reduce toxins naturally.

Use an air purifier for improved indoor air quality, particularly in bedrooms.

7. Pesticides and Herbicides

Residues on fruits, vegetables, and even lawns can introduce harmful chemicals into your system. Pesticides are known endocrine disruptors that affect thyroid function and metabolism.

Solution:

Choose organic produce whenever possible to avoid pesticide exposure.

Wash fruits and vegetables thoroughly, using a vinegar rinse for extra cleaning.

Steer clear of synthetic pesticides and herbicides when maintaining your yard.

Look for natural alternatives.

Why It Matters

Hormonal balance depends on reducing the toxic load your body faces every day. By eliminating common environmental toxins, you give your thyroid, adrenals, and entire endocrine system a chance to recover and thrive. A cleaner environment means fewer disruptions to your metabolism, energy, and mood—laying the foundation for long-term health and vitality.

Making these changes might feel overwhelming at first, but start small. Each step toward a toxin-free environment is a powerful act of self-care, and over time, these adjustments will become part of your daily routine. Remember, even small actions can lead to significant improvements in your health and energy.

Take control of your environment—because you deserve to live in a space that supports your body, mind, and well-being.

3.3 The Daily Detox Ritual: Simple Cleansing Practices

Detoxification is not just a trendy health buzzword—it's a foundational step toward hormonal balance, improved energy, and overall well-being. When your body is burdened by toxins, your thyroid, adrenal glands, and metabolism suffer, leading to fatigue, mood swings, and weight gain. A simple daily detox ritual can support your body's natural cleansing systems, helping you reset your hormones and reclaim vitality.

Why Detox Matters

Every day, your body is exposed to toxins from food, water, air, and household products. While your liver, kidneys, and lymphatic system work hard to eliminate these, a toxic overload can disrupt hormone production and lead to imbalances. Incorporating gentle detox practices into your routine can ease this burden and promote hormonal harmony.

The Morning Detox Ritual

Starting your day with detox-focused habits sets the tone for balance and clarity. Follow these steps for a simple, yet powerful cleansing routine:

1. Hydration with Warm Lemon Water
Upon waking, drink a glass of warm water with freshly squeezed lemon juice. This helps flush your liver, stimulates digestion, and alkalizes your body. Lemon water is rich in vitamin C, which supports adrenal health and boosts your immune system.

2. Dry Brushing

Before showering, use a natural bristle brush to gently exfoliate your skin in circular motions, starting from your feet and working upward. Dry brushing promotes lymphatic drainage, improves circulation, and removes dead skin cells, supporting your body's largest detox organ—your skin.

3. Gentle Movement

Engage in 10-15 minutes of light exercise like yoga, stretching, or walking. This boosts circulation, enhances lymph flow, and jumpstarts your metabolism. Gentle movement also reduces cortisol levels, helping balance your stress hormones.

4. Detoxifying Breakfast

Begin your day with a nutrient-dense breakfast such as a green smoothie or chia seed pudding. Focus on foods rich in antioxidants, fiber, and healthy fats to support liver detoxification and stabilize blood sugar.

Midday Detox Boost

The middle of the day can be an opportunity to support ongoing detoxification.

1. Stay Hydrated
Sip on water infused with cucumber, mint, or ginger to maintain hydration and encourage kidney function.

2. Mindful Breathing
Take a few moments to practice deep belly breathing. This simple act reduces stress, oxygenates your blood, and aids in toxin elimination through the lungs.

3. Eat Clean, Balanced Meals
Focus on whole foods, including leafy greens, cruciferous vegetables (like broccoli and kale), lean protein, and healthy fats. Avoid processed foods, sugar, and artificial additives, which can disrupt hormones and burden your liver.

Evening Detox Ritual

As your day winds down, your body prepares for rest and repair. These evening practices can enhance your detox efforts:

1. Epsom Salt Bath
Take a warm bath with Epsom salts to relax your muscles and draw out toxins. The magnesium in Epsom salts soothes stress and promotes better sleep, which is essential for hormone regulation.

2. Herbal Teas
Sip on calming herbal teas like chamomile, dandelion root, or milk thistle. These teas support liver detoxification, reduce bloating, and prepare your body for restful sleep.

3. Unplug and Wind Down
Reduce screen time at least an hour before bed to lower blue light exposure, which can interfere with melatonin production. Instead, practice journaling, meditation, or light reading to relax your mind and body.

Weekly Detox Practices

In addition to daily rituals, consider integrating these practices a few times a week to enhance your detox routine:

Fasting Window: Practice intermittent fasting by allowing your body a 12-16 hour break from food overnight. This gives your digestive system a chance to rest and repair.

Green Juices: Incorporate fresh, organic green juices rich in chlorophyll to cleanse your blood and boost cellular energy.

Sweat It Out: Engage in activities like sauna sessions or high-intensity exercise to promote sweating, another powerful detox pathway.

The Hormonal Reset Connection

A consistent detox ritual doesn't just cleanse your body—it creates the ideal environment for your hormones to thrive. By reducing inflammation, stabilizing blood sugar, and improving digestion, these simple practices support the delicate balance of your thyroid, adrenal glands, and reproductive hormones.

Over time, these daily habits help you feel lighter, more energized, and emotionally balanced. As you progress through The Hormone Reset Plan, these detox rituals will work hand-in-hand with the blueprint to optimize your health and transform your life.

These practices are simple, practical, and designed to fit into any lifestyle. Remember, detoxing is not about drastic measures—it's about gentle, sustainable steps that empower your body to heal naturally.

Chapter 4

Fueling Your Body with Nutrients

4.1 The Power of Anti-Inflammatory Foods

Inflammation lies at the root of many chronic health challenges, including hormonal imbalances, fatigue, weight gain, and mood disorders. The good news? Your diet is one of the most powerful tools to combat inflammation and restore balance to your body. By focusing on anti-inflammatory foods, you can naturally support your thyroid, adrenal glands, metabolism, and overall hormonal health.

Understanding Inflammation and Hormones
Inflammation is the body's inherent reaction to injury or infection. While short-term inflammation is protective, chronic inflammation wreaks havoc on the body, disrupting hormone production and signaling. Hormones like cortisol, insulin, and thyroid hormones are particularly sensitive to inflammation. This can

lead to adrenal fatigue, insulin resistance, sluggish metabolism, and imbalanced moods.

Anti-inflammatory foods work by neutralizing harmful free radicals, reducing oxidative stress, and calming the immune system. They allow your body to heal and function optimally, creating a strong foundation for hormone balance and energy restoration.

Key Anti-Inflammatory Foods to Include

1. Leafy Greens
Spinach, kale, Swiss chard, and arugula are packed with antioxidants, vitamins, and minerals like magnesium, which supports adrenal health and stabilizes mood. Leafy greens also provide chlorophyll, which helps detoxify the body and reduce inflammation.

2. Berries
Blueberries, strawberries, raspberries, and blackberries are loaded with anthocyanins—powerful antioxidants that

combat oxidative stress. Their low glycemic index also helps stabilize blood sugar, preventing insulin spikes that can disrupt hormones.

3. Fatty Fish
Salmon, mackerel, sardines, and herring are rich in omega-3 fatty acids, which reduce inflammation and support brain health. Omega-3s are particularly beneficial for improving cortisol balance and alleviating symptoms of adrenal fatigue.

4. Turmeric
This golden spice contains curcumin, a potent anti-inflammatory compound. Turmeric helps regulate cortisol levels and supports liver detoxification, which is essential for hormone metabolism. Pair it with black pepper to enhance absorption.

5. Nuts and Seeds
Almonds, walnuts, chia seeds, and flaxseeds provide healthy fats, fiber, and antioxidants.

They help regulate blood sugar and reduce inflammation, supporting overall hormonal harmony.

6. Avocado
A rich source of monounsaturated fats and vitamin E, avocado reduces inflammation and supports healthy cholesterol levels, which are crucial for hormone production.

7. Cruciferous Vegetables
Broccoli, cauliflower, Brussels sprouts, and cabbage contain compounds that promote liver detoxification and estrogen metabolism. They help prevent estrogen dominance, a common issue in hormonal imbalance.

8. Green Tea
Rich in catechins, green tea is a natural anti-inflammatory drink that boosts metabolism and supports mental clarity. It's a perfect addition to your daily routine for balancing stress hormones.

9. Ginger
Known for its warming and soothing properties, ginger reduces inflammation, aids digestion, and supports adrenal health. Add it to teas, smoothies, or stir-fries.

10. Olive Oil
Extra virgin olive oil is a staple in anti-inflammatory diets. It provides powerful antioxidants and healthy fats that support heart health, reduce inflammation, and aid in hormone production.

The Hormonal Reset Connection

In The Hormone Reset Plan, anti-inflammatory foods play a pivotal role in reducing the stress burden on your body. By calming inflammation, you're allowing your thyroid and adrenal glands to recover, boosting your metabolism and stabilizing your mood.

Each week of the 4-week blueprint focuses on incorporating these nutrient-dense foods into your meals while removing common inflammatory triggers like processed sugars, refined carbohydrates, and unhealthy fats. Over time, you'll notice reduced bloating, better energy, more stable moods, and a lighter, healthier body.

Simple Steps to Get Started

1. Start Small
Gradually replace inflammatory foods with anti-inflammatory alternatives. Swap sugary snacks for fresh berries or replace vegetable oil with olive oil.

2. Plan Ahead
Prep meals that include anti-inflammatory staples. For example, try a spinach and avocado salad topped with grilled salmon and a sprinkle of flaxseeds.

3. Hydrate with Intention

Drink green tea or ginger-infused water throughout the day to maximize anti-inflammatory benefits.

4. Stay Consistent
Remember, healing takes time. Stick with the plan, and your body will thank you with improved energy, better digestion, and balanced hormones.

Transforming Your Life, One Bite at a Time

The power of anti-inflammatory foods cannot be overstated. They are the cornerstone of hormonal health, offering a natural and sustainable way to reset your body. By embracing these healing foods, you're taking a proactive step towards reclaiming your energy, revitalizing your mood, and transforming your life.

The path to hormone balance is not about restriction—it's about nourishment. With every anti-inflammatory meal, you're giving your body the tools it needs to heal, thrive, and achieve vibrant health naturally.

4.2 Building Your Plate: A Practical Meal Guide

When striving to reset your hormones, what you eat—and how you eat it—is foundational. Your plate is more than just a vessel for food; it is a tool for nourishment, balance, and healing. Crafting meals with intention can profoundly influence your thyroid health, adrenal function, mood, and metabolism. This guide simplifies the process of building hormone-balancing meals that work seamlessly with your body's natural rhythms.

The Principles of a Balanced Plate

A hormone-friendly plate should focus on:

1. Stabilizing blood sugar

Balanced blood sugar prevents spikes and crashes, reducing stress on your adrenals and promoting consistent energy levels.

2. Supporting detox pathways

Your liver plays a critical role in hormone metabolism. A clean diet aids this process, ensuring excess hormones are eliminated effectively.

3. Providing nutrient density

Every bite counts. Choose foods that deliver vitamins, minerals, and antioxidants essential for hormone production and function.

Let's break this down into a practical meal framework.

Step 1: The Foundation—Protein (30-40% of your plate)

Protein is vital for hormone production and blood sugar stability. **Include clean, high-quality sources:**

Animal-based options: Organic chicken, pasture-raised eggs, wild-caught fish, grass-fed beef, or turkey.

Plant-based options: Lentils, quinoa, chickpeas, hemp seeds, or tofu.

Why it matters: Protein provides amino acids like tyrosine, which supports thyroid hormone production, and helps build neurotransmitters for a balanced mood.

Step 2: The Centerpiece—Non-Starchy Vegetables (40-50% of your plate)

Vegetables provide fiber, antioxidants, and essential nutrients to support detoxification and gut health, which are critical for hormone balance. **Focus on a variety of colors:**

Cruciferous vegetables: Broccoli, kale, Brussels sprouts, and cauliflower support estrogen detoxification.

Leafy greens: Spinach, arugula, and Swiss chard provide magnesium, crucial for stress regulation and adrenal health.

Other favorites: Bell peppers, zucchini, asparagus, or mushrooms for added phytonutrients.

Pro tip: Aim for half your plate to be vegetables, lightly steamed, roasted, or raw, to preserve nutrients.

Step 3: The Energy Source—Healthy Fats (20-25% of your plate)

Fats are the building blocks of hormone production and aid in absorbing fat-soluble vitamins like A, D, E, and K. **Include:**

✓ Avocados

✓ Olive oil

✓ Coconut oil

✓ Nuts and seeds (almonds, flaxseeds, chia seeds)

✓ Fatty fish (salmon, mackerel, sardines)

Why it matters: Healthy fats stabilize blood sugar, reduce inflammation, and provide precursors for hormone synthesis.

Step 4: Optional Additions—Complex Carbohydrates (10-20% of your plate)

While not always necessary, complex carbohydrates can be helpful, especially if you are dealing with adrenal fatigue or low energy. **Choose:**

✓ Sweet potatoes

✓ Quinoa

✓ Brown rice

✓ Legumes

Note: Keep portion sizes moderate to avoid blood sugar spikes, especially if you have insulin resistance or weight loss goals.

Step 5: Flavor and Function—Herbs, Spices, and Fermented Foods

Enhance your meals with healing flavors:

Spices: Turmeric, cinnamon, and ginger reduce inflammation and support metabolism.

Herbs: Basil, cilantro, and parsley are rich in antioxidants.

Fermented foods: Sauerkraut, kimchi, or yogurt improve gut health, aiding hormone regulation.

Building a Day of Balanced Meals

Breakfast:

Scrambled pasture-raised eggs with sautéed spinach and avocado slices.

A side of fermented sauerkraut for gut health.

Lunch:

Grilled chicken breast over a bed of mixed greens, shredded carrots, and cucumbers, dressed with olive oil and lemon juice.

A small serving of quinoa for sustained energy.

Dinner:

Baked wild-caught salmon with roasted Brussels sprouts and mashed cauliflower.

Sprinkle with turmeric and black pepper for added anti-inflammatory benefits.

Hydration: An Often Overlooked Component

Hydration is crucial for hormone balance. Drink plenty of water, herbal teas, or infused water with lemon, cucumber, or mint. Avoid sugary drinks and excessive caffeine, which can stress your adrenals.

Adjusting for Your Unique Needs

Every individual is different, and your plate should reflect your specific goals and challenges. Experiment with portions and foods to discover what makes you feel energized, focused, and balanced.

By thoughtfully building your plate, you're not just eating to satisfy hunger; you're creating a daily practice of self-care and hormone harmony. Small, intentional changes to your meals can lead to profound transformations in your energy, mood, and overall well-being. Start today, and let every meal bring you closer to reclaiming your health.

4.3 Hormone-Boosting Smoothies and Beverages

Nourishing your body with hormone-friendly ingredients is a powerful way to restore balance and energy. Below are recipes designed to support your thyroid, adrenal health, mood, and metabolism using natural ingredients.

1. Adrenal Support Smoothie

This smoothie helps calm stress and nourish adrenal glands with adaptogens and healthy fats.

Ingredients:

• 1 cup of plain almond milk (or any nut milk of your choice).

• 1 small banana (frozen for creaminess)

• 1 tablespoon almond butter

- 1 teaspoon maca powder (supports adrenal balance)

- 1 teaspoon raw cacao powder (boosts mood and reduces stress)

- 1/4 teaspoon cinnamon (balances blood sugar)

- 1 scoop protein powder (optional for added nutrition)

- A handful of ice

Instructions:

1. Add all ingredients to a blender.

2. Blend on high until smooth and creamy.

3. Pour into a glass and enjoy as a morning or afternoon pick-me-up.

2. Thyroid-Loving Green Smoothie

Rich in nutrients that support thyroid function and detoxification.

Ingredients:

- 1 cup coconut water (hydrating and rich in electrolytes)

- 1/2 avocado (provides healthy fats for hormone production)

- 1 handful spinach or kale (loaded with thyroid-friendly nutrients like magnesium)

- 1/4 cup pineapple (supports digestion and anti-inflammatory effects)

- 1 tablespoon ground flaxseeds (a source of omega-3s and fiber)

- Juice of 1/2 lemon (aids detoxification)

• A small piece of fresh ginger (optional for digestion and inflammation)

Instructions:

1. Place all ingredients into a blender.

2. Blend until smooth, adding water if needed for consistency.

3. Drink immediately to maximize freshness and nutrient benefits.

3. Hormone Harmony Golden Milk

This soothing, warm beverage reduces inflammation and supports overall hormonal balance.

Ingredients:

• 1 cup unsweetened coconut milk (rich in medium-chain triglycerides for energy)

- 1/2 teaspoon turmeric powder (anti-inflammatory and hormone-balancing)

- 1/4 teaspoon cinnamon (regulates blood sugar)

- 1/8 teaspoon black pepper (enhances turmeric absorption)

- 1 teaspoon raw honey (optional for sweetness)

- 1/2 teaspoon ghee or coconut oil (supports fat-soluble vitamin absorption)

Instructions:

1. In a small saucepan, heat coconut milk over low heat.

2. Stir in turmeric, cinnamon, black pepper, and ghee.

3. Whisk well until heated through (do not boil).

4. Sweeten with honey if desired.

5. Pour into a mug and enjoy before bed for relaxation.

4. Metabolism-Boosting Berry Smoothie

Rich in antioxidants and nutrients that promote energy and enhance metabolism.

Ingredients:

•1 cup water or unsweetened almond milk

•1/2 cup frozen mixed berries (blueberries, raspberries, strawberries)

•1/2 small beet (boosts blood flow and energy)

•1 tablespoon chia seeds (provides fiber and omega-3s)

•1 teaspoon apple cider vinegar (stimulates digestion)

- 1 scoop collagen powder (supports skin, hair, and joint health)

- A handful of ice

Instructions:

1. Blend all ingredients until smooth.

2. Adjust sweetness with a bit of stevia or honey, if needed.

3. Pour into a glass and enjoy as a refreshing snack or meal replacement.

5. Mood-Boosting Herbal Tea

A calming tea blend to reduce anxiety and promote emotional well-being.

Ingredients:

- 1 cup hot water

- 1 teaspoon dried chamomile flowers

- 1 teaspoon dried lavender buds

- 1 teaspoon dried lemon balm (optional)

- 1/2 teaspoon raw honey (optional)

Instructions:

1. Combine chamomile, lavender, and lemon balm in a tea infuser or teapot.

2. Pour hot water over the herbs and let steep for 5-7 minutes.

3. Strain, sweeten with honey if desired, and sip slowly.

These beverages are simple yet powerful tools to nourish your body and reset your hormones naturally. Incorporate them into your daily routine for lasting energy, balance, and vitality.

Week 2: Rebuild and Stabilize

Chapter 5

Stabilizing Blood Sugar and Insulin

5.1 The Blood Sugar-Hormone Connection

Blood sugar balance is one of the most critical, yet often overlooked, components of hormonal health. Our bodies are finely tuned systems where hormones like insulin, cortisol, and sex hormones work together to maintain balance. When blood sugar levels spike or crash, this harmony is disrupted, leading to a cascade of effects that impact your thyroid, adrenals, mood, and metabolism.

In The Hormone Reset Plan, we take a closer look at how stabilizing blood sugar levels can be a game-changer for reclaiming energy, improving mood, and restoring hormonal balance. This connection forms the foundation of your 4-week blueprint to reset and revitalize your body naturally.

How Blood Sugar Impacts Hormones

1. Insulin: The Gatekeeper of Energy

Insulin is a hormone released by your pancreas to regulate blood sugar levels. When you consume carbohydrates or sugar, insulin helps transport glucose into your cells for energy. However, consuming too many processed foods, sugary snacks, or skipping meals can lead to insulin spikes and crashes. Over time, this can result in insulin resistance—a condition where your cells stop responding to insulin effectively. This resistance not only disrupts blood sugar balance but also affects your body's ability to regulate other hormones.

2. Cortisol: The Stress Hormone

When your blood sugar drops too low (hypoglycemia), your body perceives it as a stressor. In response, your adrenal glands release cortisol to help stabilize your blood sugar by signaling the liver to release stored glucose. However, frequent blood sugar crashes can lead to chronic cortisol elevation. High cortisol levels disrupt sleep, increase belly fat, and negatively affect thyroid and sex hormones.

3. Thyroid Hormones: The Metabolic Regulators

Unbalanced blood sugar can strain your thyroid. Insulin resistance and high cortisol levels can impair the conversion of T4 (inactive thyroid hormone) into T3 (active thyroid hormone), slowing your metabolism and leading to fatigue, weight gain, and mood disturbances.

4. Sex Hormones: Estrogen, Progesterone, and Testosterone

Blood sugar fluctuations also impact estrogen, progesterone, and testosterone levels. Insulin resistance can cause your ovaries to produce more testosterone, contributing to conditions like polycystic ovary syndrome (PCOS). Additionally, high cortisol levels can reduce progesterone, which is essential for mood stability and reproductive health.

The Role of Diet in Balancing Blood Sugar and Hormones

Diet plays a pivotal role in maintaining stable blood sugar levels and supporting hormonal balance. **Here's how you can make small but powerful changes:**

Choose Whole Foods Over Processed Foods
Opt for nutrient-dense whole foods, such as vegetables, lean proteins, healthy fats, and whole grains. These foods provide steady energy and prevent blood sugar spikes.

Prioritize Protein and Healthy Fats
Incorporate protein and healthy fats into every meal. They slow down glucose absorption, keeping your blood sugar stable and reducing cravings. **Examples** include eggs, nuts, seeds, avocados, and fatty fish.

Avoid Sugary Snacks
Eliminate refined sugars and high-glycemic foods like sodas, pastries, and white bread.

Replace them with natural sweeteners like honey or fruits with fiber, such as berries.

Eat Balanced Meals Regularly
Skipping meals can lead to blood sugar crashes. Stick to regular eating times and ensure every meal includes a balance of macronutrients.

Lifestyle Strategies to Support Blood Sugar and Hormonal Health

1. Exercise Wisely
Engage in regular physical activity to improve insulin sensitivity. Strength training and moderate-intensity cardio are particularly effective. Avoid overtraining, as excessive exercise can elevate cortisol levels.

2. Practice Stress Management
Chronic stress can wreak havoc on your hormones. Incorporate stress-reducing practices like deep breathing, meditation, or yoga to help regulate cortisol and stabilize blood sugar.

3. Prioritize Sleep

Poor sleep disrupts blood sugar regulation and increases cortisol. Aim for 7–9 hours of quality sleep each night by maintaining a consistent bedtime routine.

Reset Your Body in 4 Weeks

This 4-week blueprint outlined in The Hormone Reset Plan will guide you in stabilizing your blood sugar, supporting your thyroid, calming your adrenals, and rebalancing your sex hormones. By addressing blood sugar at its core, you'll unlock the energy, clarity, and balance your body craves.

Each week, you'll implement small, actionable steps to create lasting change. From meal planning tips to lifestyle tweaks, this plan is designed to be practical and effective. By the end of the four weeks, you'll feel empowered to take control of your hormonal health naturally and sustainably.

Take the first step today—balance your blood sugar, and watch your body transform. Reclaim your energy, uplift your mood, and enjoy the vibrant health you deserve!

5.2 Balanced Meals: Combining Protein, Fat, and Fiber

Creating balanced meals is a cornerstone of The Hormone Reset Plan. By focusing on a thoughtful combination of protein, fat, and fiber, you can support your body's natural hormonal rhythms, stabilize blood sugar levels, and fuel your energy reserves. **Let's explore why these three macronutrients matter and how to bring them together for meals that nourish and heal.**

Why Protein, Fat, and Fiber?

1. Protein:
Protein is the building block of every cell in your body. It supports muscle repair, stabilizes blood sugar, and plays a key role in the production of hormones like insulin, which regulates energy.

Adequate protein also helps manage cravings by increasing satiety, keeping you full longer.

Examples: Organic eggs, wild-caught fish, grass-fed meats, lentils, and quinoa.

2. Healthy Fats:
Far from being the enemy, healthy fats are essential for hormonal balance. They provide the raw materials for making hormones like estrogen and testosterone, reduce inflammation, and keep your brain sharp. Healthy fats also help your body absorb fat-soluble vitamins (A, D, E, and K).

Examples: Avocados, olive oil, nuts, seeds, and fatty fish like salmon.

3. Fiber:
Fiber is your digestive system's best friend. It slows the absorption of sugar into the bloodstream, helping to prevent insulin spikes. Fiber also feeds your gut microbiome, which

influences everything from digestion to mood and hormone regulation.

Examples: Leafy greens, berries, flaxseeds, chia seeds, and whole grains like oats.

How to Combine These Macronutrients

To create a truly balanced meal, include all three components—protein, fat, and fiber—in the right proportions. This balance keeps your blood sugar stable, prevents energy crashes, and supports healthy metabolism.

Here's how to build your plate:

1. Start with Protein:

Choose a palm-sized portion of lean protein for meals, like grilled chicken, tofu, or tempeh.

For snacks, try a boiled egg, a handful of almonds, or Greek yogurt.

2. Add Healthy Fats:

Use 1-2 tablespoons of healthy fats per meal. Drizzle olive oil over your salad or add a dollop of almond butter to your morning smoothie.

Snack on small portions of nuts, seeds, or olives for an energy boost.

3. Fill Up on Fiber:

Fill at least half your plate with fiber-rich vegetables, such as broccoli, spinach, or zucchini.

Include high-fiber carbs like sweet potatoes, lentils, or quinoa in smaller portions for sustained energy.

Sample Meal Ideas

1. Breakfast:

Scrambled eggs cooked in coconut oil, served with sautéed spinach and half an avocado.

A smoothie with Greek yogurt, a handful of mixed berries, spinach, chia seeds, and almond butter.

2. Lunch:

Grilled salmon on a bed of leafy greens, topped with sunflower seeds and drizzled with olive oil and lemon juice.

Lentil soup with a side of sliced cucumbers and hummus.

3. Dinner:

Grass-fed beef or plant-based protein served with roasted sweet potatoes and steamed asparagus, drizzled with tahini sauce.

Baked chicken breast with quinoa and sautéed kale in garlic and avocado oil.

4. Snacks:

Apple slices with almond butter.

Handful of walnuts paired with fresh cucumber slices.

Benefits of Balanced Meals

1. Stable Energy: Balanced meals prevent the rollercoaster of energy spikes and crashes that often lead to fatigue.

2. Reduced Cravings: Combining protein, fat, and fiber ensures you're satisfied and less likely to overindulge.

3. Improved Hormone Health: These macronutrients work together to support the production, regulation, and balance of essential hormones.

4. Enhanced Metabolism: A steady intake of nutrient-rich meals keeps your metabolism functioning at its best.

By prioritizing protein, healthy fats, and fiber in every meal, you empower your body to reset and thrive. This simple yet powerful approach is at the heart of The Hormone Reset Plan—helping you reclaim your energy, stabilize your mood, and revitalize your thyroid, adrenals, and metabolism naturally.

5.3 Snack Smart: Easy, Hormone-Friendly Snacks

Balancing hormones naturally requires nourishing your body with the right snacks that stabilize blood sugar, support your thyroid and adrenals, and provide essential nutrients for energy and mood. These easy, hormone-friendly snack recipes are designed to fit seamlessly into your lifestyle. They are rich in whole, clean ingredients and crafted to help you feel your best during the journey to hormonal balance.

1. Almond-Avocado Protein Bites

Ingredients

- 1 cup raw almonds (soaked overnight and drained)
- 1 ripe avocado
- 2 tablespoons chia seeds
- 1 tablespoon flaxseed meal
- 1 tablespoon raw honey (optional)
- ½ teaspoon cinnamon
- 1 teaspoon vanilla extract
- Pinch of sea salt

Instructions

1. Blend almonds in a food processor until finely chopped.

2. Add avocado, chia seeds, flaxseed meal, honey, cinnamon, vanilla extract, and sea salt. Blend until the mixture becomes dough-like.

3. Roll into bite-sized balls and refrigerate for 1 hour before serving.

4. Keep refrigerated in a sealed container and use within 5 days.

Benefits: Almonds and flaxseeds provide hormone-supporting healthy fats, while chia seeds stabilize blood sugar for steady energy.

2. Sweet Potato and Hummus Bites

Ingredients

- 1 large sweet potato (sliced into ¼-inch rounds)

- ½ cup hummus (plain or flavored)

- 1 tablespoon extra virgin olive oil
- 1 teaspoon smoked paprika
- Fresh parsley for garnish

Instructions

1. Preheat the oven to 400°F (200°C). Arrange sweet potato slices on a baking sheet lined with parchment paper.

2. Drizzle olive oil over the slices and sprinkle with smoked paprika. Roast for 20–25 minutes, flipping halfway through.

3. Once cooled, top each slice with a dollop of hummus and garnish with fresh parsley.

4. Serve immediately or store sweet potato slices in an airtight container and add hummus before eating.

Benefits: Sweet potatoes are a great source of slow-digesting carbohydrates and vitamin A, which supports adrenal function.

3. Hormone-Balancing Smoothie Bowl

Ingredients

- 1 cup unsweetened almond milk

- ½ frozen banana

- 1 handful spinach

- ½ cup frozen mixed berries

- 1 scoop plant-based protein powder (optional)

- 1 tablespoon almond butter

- 1 tablespoon ground flaxseeds

- 1 teaspoon maca powder

Toppings: sliced almonds, chia seeds, shredded coconut

Instructions

1. Combine almond milk, banana, spinach, berries, protein powder, almond butter, flaxseeds, and maca powder in a blender. Blend until smooth.

2. Pour into a bowl and top with your favorite hormone-friendly toppings.

3. Serve immediately.

Benefits: Maca powder supports energy and mood, while flaxseeds provide phytoestrogens to balance estrogen levels.

4. Turmeric Pumpkin Seed Trail Mix

Ingredients

- 1 cup raw pumpkin seeds

- ½ cup raw walnuts

- ¼ cup dried cranberries (unsweetened)

- 1 tablespoon coconut oil

- 1 teaspoon turmeric powder

- ½ teaspoon sea salt

- ¼ teaspoon black pepper

Instructions

1. In a skillet, heat coconut oil over medium heat. Add pumpkin seeds and walnuts.

2. Sprinkle with turmeric powder, sea salt, and black pepper. Toast for 5–7 minutes, stirring constantly, until golden and fragrant.

3. Remove from heat and mix in dried cranberries.

4. Let cool before storing in an airtight container.

Benefits: Pumpkin seeds and walnuts are rich in zinc and magnesium, essential for hormone production and adrenal health.

5. Greek Yogurt Berry Parfait

Ingredients

- ½ cup unsweetened Greek yogurt (or coconut yogurt for dairy-free)

- ¼ cup fresh mixed berries (blueberries, raspberries, blackberries)

- 1 tablespoon hemp seeds

- 1 teaspoon raw honey or maple syrup

Instructions

1. Layer Greek yogurt and berries in a glass or bowl.

2. Sprinkle with hemp seeds and drizzle with honey or maple syrup.

3. Enjoy immediately.

Benefits: Greek yogurt supports gut health with probiotics, which play a key role in hormone balance.

These snacks are perfect to support your journey toward hormone health. They stabilize your energy, reduce cravings, and provide essential nutrients for thyroid, adrenal, and metabolic balance.

Chapter 6

Gentle Movement and Stress Relief

6.1 Exercises That Balance Hormones

Exercise plays a powerful role in balancing hormones, helping to regulate systems throughout the body and restore overall harmony. The right types of movement can reduce stress, boost energy, and promote better sleep—key factors in resetting your hormones. When you focus on exercises that specifically target hormone balance, you can revitalize your thyroid, support adrenal function, improve your mood, and enhance metabolism. This approach is particularly transformative when paired with a structured plan like The Hormone Reset Plan.

In this unique four-week blueprint, exercise is a cornerstone of natural hormone restoration. **Below are the key types of exercises that promote hormonal balance and how to incorporate them into your life effectively.**

1. Low-Intensity Movement for Stress Reduction

Chronic stress leads to elevated cortisol levels, which can disrupt sleep, thyroid function, and weight management. Low-intensity exercises like walking, yoga, and stretching are excellent for lowering cortisol and promoting relaxation.

Why it works: Gentle movement helps activate the parasympathetic nervous system, often called the "rest-and-digest" system, which counterbalances the stress response.

How to start: Aim for 30–60 minutes of low-impact movement daily. A morning walk outdoors can be particularly calming and energizing.

2. Strength Training for Better Metabolism and Insulin Sensitivity

Building muscle through strength training boosts your metabolism and helps regulate insulin, a key hormone involved in blood sugar control. Resistance exercises also stimulate the release of growth hormone, which supports tissue repair and overall vitality.

Why it works: Strong muscles improve how your body processes glucose, reducing the risk of insulin resistance—a common issue linked to hormonal imbalances like PCOS or type 2 diabetes.

How to start: Incorporate 2–3 sessions of strength training each week, focusing on full-body exercises such as squats, lunges, and push-ups. Use body weight, resistance bands, or light dumbbells to start.

3. High-Intensity Interval Training (HIIT) for Fat Burning

Short bursts of intense exercise followed by rest can help balance hormones related to fat storage, such as insulin and cortisol. HIIT also triggers the release of endorphins, improving mood and reducing symptoms of depression or anxiety.

Why it works: HIIT can stimulate the production of adiponectin, a hormone that regulates fat metabolism, while minimizing the risk of overtraining, which can spike cortisol.

How to start: Try 20–30 minutes of interval training 1–2 times a week. Alternate 30 seconds of high effort (e.g., sprinting or jumping jacks) with 1–2 minutes of low-intensity recovery.

4. Pelvic Floor and Core Exercises for Hormonal Balance in Women

For women, the pelvic floor plays a critical role in hormonal health, particularly after childbirth or during menopause. Core-strengthening exercises like Pilates or targeted pelvic floor work can enhance circulation, reduce inflammation, and support reproductive health.

Why it works: A healthy pelvic floor improves blood flow to the ovaries and adrenal glands, which produce key hormones like estrogen and progesterone.

How to start: Practice 10–15 minutes of pelvic floor exercises daily, such as Kegels, bridges, or gentle core strengthening moves.

5. Mind-Body Exercises for Emotional and Hormonal Health

Stress and emotional imbalances often lead to disruptions in hormone production. Practices like tai chi, qigong, or mindful yoga combine movement with deep breathing, helping to reduce stress, lower cortisol, and improve overall well-being.

Why it works: These exercises support the hypothalamic-pituitary-adrenal (HPA) axis, the body's central stress-response system.

How to start: Dedicate 15–20 minutes each day to a mind-body practice. Evening sessions can be especially helpful for promoting restful sleep.

6. Regular Stretching and Flexibility Work to Enhance Circulation

Stretching improves blood flow, delivering oxygen and nutrients to hormone-producing glands like the thyroid, adrenal glands, and ovaries. Enhanced circulation helps regulate hormone levels and promotes detoxification.

Why it works: Stretching also releases physical tension, which can prevent the body from slipping into a chronic stress state.

How to start: Spend 10–15 minutes stretching major muscle groups, focusing on deep, slow breaths to enhance relaxation.

Building Your 4-Week Hormone Reset Plan

Incorporate a balanced mix of these exercises into your weekly routine for optimal results. **Here's a suggested framework:**

Day 1: Strength training + 20-minute walk

Day 2: Mindful yoga or tai chi

Day 3: HIIT session + core strengthening

Day 4: Low-intensity stretching or a gentle hike

Day 5: Strength training

Day 6: Pelvic floor exercises + a calming walk

Day 7: Rest or restorative yoga

By committing to these exercises, you'll not only balance your hormones but also reclaim your energy, improve your mood, and boost your metabolism. This simple yet effective approach supports your body's natural ability to heal and thrive. When combined with the other strategies outlined in The Hormone Reset Plan, this exercise routine becomes a powerful tool for transformation.

6.2 The Art of Stress Management: Mindfulness and Relaxation

Stress is an inevitable part of life, but how we respond to it can make all the difference in our physical and emotional health. Mindfulness and relaxation are two powerful tools that can transform how we experience stress, allowing us to navigate challenges with calm and resilience.

Understanding Stress and Its Impact

Stress is more than just a feeling—it's a physical and emotional response to demands or pressures. While short-term stress can motivate and focus us, chronic stress wreaks havoc on the body, disrupting hormones, impairing the immune system, and contributing to anxiety, fatigue, and even weight gain. Managing stress effectively is essential, particularly when working to reset the delicate balance of your body's hormones.

Why Mindfulness Matters

Mindfulness is the practice of staying present in the moment, observing thoughts and feelings without judgment. It teaches you to focus your attention and become aware of the connection between your mind and body. Regular mindfulness practice can reduce cortisol, the stress hormone, and improve overall well-being.

Simple ways to incorporate mindfulness into daily life include:

1. Mindful Breathing: Take slow, deep breaths, focusing on the sensation of air entering and leaving your lungs.

2. Body Scans: Gradually bring attention to different parts of your body, releasing tension as you go.

3. Mindful Observation: Notice the details of your surroundings—colors, textures, sounds—grounding yourself in the present moment.

Relaxation Techniques for Stress Relief

Relaxation techniques counteract the stress response, helping the body return to a state of rest and balance. **Here are a few effective methods:**

1. Progressive Muscle Relaxation: Tense and relax each muscle group, starting at your toes and working upward. This helps release physical tension while calming the mind.

2. Guided Imagery: Close your eyes and visualize a peaceful scene, such as a beach or forest, immersing yourself in the details to foster relaxation.

3. Yoga and Stretching: Gentle movement paired with deep breathing improves circulation, reduces muscle tension, and calms the nervous system.

4. Meditation: Set aside a few minutes daily to sit quietly, focus on your breath, and let go of distracting thoughts.

Integrating Mindfulness and Relaxation into the Hormone Reset Plan

Stress management is a cornerstone of restoring hormonal balance. Chronic stress overloads the adrenal glands, leading to cortisol imbalances that disrupt your thyroid, metabolism, and mood. **Incorporating mindfulness and relaxation into your 4-week blueprint for hormone health can:**

✓ Stabilize cortisol levels, reducing stress-induced weight gain.

✓ Support thyroid and adrenal function, restoring energy.

✓ Improve sleep quality, enhancing mood and overall health.

Begin by dedicating 10–15 minutes each day to mindfulness or relaxation practices. Gradually increase the time as these practices become habits. Pairing stress management with a hormone-supportive diet, gentle exercise, and adequate rest creates a holistic foundation for healing.

Transforming Stress into Strength

Stress doesn't have to control your life. By embracing mindfulness and relaxation, you can retrain your mind and body to respond to challenges with grace and composure. As you progress through The Hormone Reset Plan, you'll not only rebalance your hormones but also cultivate a sense of inner peace and resilience that will serve you long after the 4-week plan is complete.

Remember, the art of stress management is not about eliminating stress but learning to dance with it—turning what once felt overwhelming into an opportunity for growth, balance, and transformation.

6.3 Restoring Energy with Adaptogens

In the journey to reclaim energy and restore balance, adaptogens play a pivotal role. These remarkable, plant-based substances help your body adapt to stress, improve resilience, and support overall hormonal harmony. They work by modulating your body's stress response, stabilizing cortisol levels, and enhancing energy reserves—all crucial for revitalizing the thyroid, adrenals, mood, and metabolism.

What Are Adaptogens?

Adaptogens are natural substances derived from herbs and mushrooms. They earned their name for their unique ability to "adapt" to your body's needs. Unlike stimulants that provide a temporary energy boost, adaptogens work at a deeper level, supporting and regulating your stress response systems. They don't overstimulate or suppress but instead bring balance, fostering long-term vitality.

The Role of Stress in Hormonal Imbalance

Stress is one of the most significant contributors to hormonal dysfunction. Chronic stress keeps your adrenal glands in overdrive, leading to excess cortisol production. Over time, this can disrupt the delicate interplay of hormones, leaving you fatigued, irritable, and struggling with weight gain or mood swings. Adaptogens act as allies, helping your body to recover from and resist the harmful effects of stress.

Key Adaptogens for Energy and Hormonal Balance

1. Ashwagandha

A star player in Ayurvedic medicine, ashwagandha supports the adrenal glands by reducing cortisol levels and enhancing your body's ability to handle stress. Studies have shown it can improve energy, reduce anxiety, and even support thyroid function, making it a top choice for restoring hormonal balance.

2. Rhodiola Rosea

Known for its ability to combat fatigue and enhance mental clarity, Rhodiola is a favorite for those battling burnout. It boosts energy by improving mitochondrial function—the powerhouse of your cells—and reduces oxidative stress, a key factor in hormonal imbalance.

3. Holy Basil (Tulsi)

This revered herb is celebrated for its calming effects and ability to lower stress hormones. Holy basil not only balances cortisol but also supports blood sugar levels, which is crucial for maintaining steady energy throughout the day.

4. Maca Root

Native to Peru, maca root is well-known for enhancing stamina, libido, and mood. It acts as a natural endocrine system balancer, nourishing the hypothalamus and pituitary glands to improve overall hormonal function.

5. Eleuthero (Siberian Ginseng)

This adaptogen is a powerhouse for improving physical endurance and mental focus. Eleuthero strengthens your adrenal glands, helping you adapt to physical and emotional stress while promoting sustained energy levels.

How to Incorporate Adaptogens into Your Routine

1. Start with a Single Adaptogen

Introduce one adaptogen at a time to understand how your body responds. Begin with a small dose, gradually increasing as needed.

2. Use High-Quality Products

Choose organic, sustainably sourced adaptogens to ensure maximum efficacy. Look for powders, teas, capsules, or tinctures that suit your lifestyle.

3. Pair with a Balanced Diet

Adaptogens work best when combined with nutrient-dense foods. Focus on whole grains, lean proteins, healthy fats, and a variety of colorful fruits and vegetables to provide a strong foundation for your hormonal health.

4. Stay Consistent

Consistency is key. Incorporate adaptogens daily for at least 4-6 weeks to experience noticeable benefits.

A 4-Week Blueprint to Restore Energy

Week 1: Balance Stress with Ashwagandha.

Take ashwagandha in the evening to promote relaxation and better sleep while reducing cortisol.

Week 2: Boost Energy with Rhodiola.
Add Rhodiola to your morning routine to combat fatigue and enhance focus. Pair it with a healthy breakfast rich in protein and fiber.

Week 3: Enhance Stability with Holy Basil.
Sip on holy basil tea throughout the day to support your adrenals and stabilize blood sugar.

Week 4: Elevate Stamina with Maca
Incorporate maca powder into smoothies or oatmeal for an energizing start to your day.

The Power of Adaptogens in Hormonal Health

Adaptogens are more than just herbs; they're a lifeline for modern living. They don't promise overnight miracles but offer sustainable, long-term benefits by addressing the root causes of fatigue and hormonal imbalance. When integrated into a comprehensive plan like The Hormone Reset Plan, adaptogens can help you reclaim your energy, reset your body, and transform your life—naturally and effectively.

By working with your body's innate ability to heal and adapt, these natural allies pave the way for renewed vitality, emotional stability, and lasting wellness.

Week 3: Restore and Recharge

Chapter 7

Supporting Thyroid and Adrenal Health

7.1 Foods and Nutrients for Thyroid Support

The thyroid gland is a small but powerful organ that plays a critical role in regulating your metabolism, energy levels, mood, and overall well-being. Supporting your thyroid naturally through nutrition is one of the most effective ways to restore balance and vitality. Here, we'll explore foods rich in key nutrients your thyroid thrives on and provide practical, easy-to-follow steps to incorporate them into your daily diet.

Key Nutrients for Thyroid Health

1. Iodine

Essential for the production of thyroid hormones.

Sources: Seaweed (nori, kelp, wakame), iodized salt, dairy products, and fish like cod and tuna.

2. Selenium

Supports thyroid hormone conversion and protects against oxidative damage.

Sources: Brazil nuts, sunflower seeds, sardines, eggs, and mushrooms.

3. Zinc

Crucial for thyroid hormone synthesis and immune function.

Sources: Pumpkin seeds, chickpeas, cashews, beef, and poultry.

4. Vitamin D

Regulates immune function and supports thyroid health.

Sources: Fatty fish (salmon, mackerel), fortified foods, egg yolks, and sunlight exposure.

5. Iron

Vital for efficient thyroid hormone production.

Sources: Spinach, lentils, red meat, quinoa, and tofu.

6. Tyrosine

An amino acid necessary for thyroid hormone synthesis.

Sources: Chicken, turkey, fish, dairy, nuts, and beans.

7. Omega-3 Fatty Acids

Reduce inflammation and support thyroid and hormonal balance.

Sources: Chia seeds, flaxseeds, walnuts, and fatty fish.

Thyroid-Supporting Foods

Breakfast: Thyroid-Boosting Smoothie

Ingredients:

- 1 cup unsweetened almond milk

- 1 cup spinach (rich in iron)

- 1 small banana (natural sweetness)

- 1 tablespoon chia seeds (omega-3 source)

- 2 Brazil nuts (selenium powerhouse)

- 1 scoop collagen powder (source of tyrosine)

- Ice cubes (optional)

Instructions:

1. Blend all ingredients until smooth.

2. Serve immediately for a nutrient-dense start to your day.

Lunch: Wild Salmon Salad with Spinach

Ingredients:

- 4 oz wild-caught salmon (omega-3 and vitamin D source)

- 2 cups fresh spinach (iron-rich greens)

- 1/2 avocado (healthy fats)

- 1 tablespoon pumpkin seeds (zinc-packed)

- 1/2 lemon (for dressing)

- A drizzle of extra virgin olive oil

Instructions:

1. Grill or bake salmon with a pinch of salt and pepper.

2. Toss spinach, avocado, and pumpkin seeds in a bowl.

3. Add the grilled salmon and drizzle with olive oil and lemon juice.

Dinner: Seaweed and Vegetable Stir-Fry

Ingredients:

- 1 sheet of nori, shredded (iodine-rich)

- 1 cup broccoli florets (supports detoxification)

- 1/2 cup mushrooms (selenium source)

- 1 small carrot, sliced

- 1 tablespoon coconut aminos (low-sodium soy sauce alternative)

- 1 teaspoon sesame oil

- 1/2 cup cooked quinoa (iron-rich grain)

Instructions:

1. Heat sesame oil in a pan and sauté broccoli, mushrooms, and carrots until tender.

2. Add shredded nori and stir in coconut aminos.

3. Serve over cooked quinoa for a nourishing dinner.

Snack: Selenium-Rich Trail Mix

Ingredients:

- 1/4 cup Brazil nuts

- 1/4 cup sunflower seeds

- 1/4 cup dried cranberries (unsweetened)

- 1/4 cup dark chocolate chips (70% or higher cacao)

Instructions:

1. Mix all ingredients in a bowl.

2. Store in an airtight container for a grab-and-go snack.

Tips for Long-Term Thyroid Health

Stay Hydrated: Drink plenty of filtered water to support detoxification and hormone balance.

Limit Goitrogens: Cook cruciferous vegetables (like kale, cauliflower, and Brussels sprouts) to reduce compounds that may interfere with thyroid function.

Avoid Processed Foods: Minimize refined sugars and artificial additives that can disrupt hormones.

Include Probiotics: Support gut health with fermented foods like yogurt, kefir, sauerkraut, or a high-quality probiotic supplement.

By consistently choosing thyroid-supportive foods, you can create a foundation for healing and restore the energy, clarity, and vitality you deserve. This approach integrates seamlessly into The Hormone Reset Plan, enabling you to reclaim your health naturally in just four weeks.

7.2 Replenishing Adrenal Reserves Naturally
Adrenal glands, often called the body's stress managers, play a pivotal role in regulating hormones that govern energy, mood, metabolism, and even immune response. Chronic stress, poor diet, lack of sleep, and exposure to environmental toxins can deplete these reserves, leaving you feeling fatigued, irritable, and out of balance. Replenishing adrenal reserves naturally is a transformative process that allows you to regain vitality and

energy while supporting long-term hormonal health.

In The Hormone Reset Plan, we focus on a unique, practical, and effective 4-week blueprint to restore adrenal health. By addressing the root causes of adrenal fatigue and adopting sustainable lifestyle changes, you can rejuvenate your adrenal function and bring balance back to your body. **Here's how to get started.**

1. Nourish Your Adrenals with Targeted Nutrition

The food you eat can either deplete or replenish your adrenal glands. **To rebuild adrenal reserves:**

Prioritize Whole, Nutrient-Dense Foods: Incorporate high-quality proteins, healthy fats, and complex carbohydrates. These stabilize blood sugar levels, preventing energy crashes that stress your adrenals.

Add Adaptogenic Herbs: Ashwagandha, holy basil, and rhodiola rosea are powerful adaptogens that support stress resilience and adrenal recovery.

Hydrate with Electrolyte-Rich Beverages: Coconut water, herbal teas, and water with a pinch of sea salt help maintain the mineral balance your adrenals need to function optimally.

Limit Stimulants and Processed Foods: Caffeine, refined sugars, and heavily processed foods strain the adrenal glands, so reducing these is key to recovery.

2. Rebalance with Restorative Sleep

Quality sleep is essential for adrenal repair. Strive to get between 7 and 9 hours of continuous sleep every night.

Create a calming bedtime routine that might include:

Turning off screens at least an hour before bed.

Practicing deep breathing or meditation to signal to your body that it's time to rest.

Keeping your bedroom dark, cool, and free from distractions to support melatonin production.

3. Manage Stress with Intentional Practices

Chronic stress is a major contributor to adrenal fatigue. Adopting stress-reducing habits can profoundly impact your recovery. **Some effective techniques include:**

Mindfulness and Meditation: Even 10 minutes a day can lower cortisol levels and improve adrenal health.

Yoga and Gentle Movement: Low-impact exercises promote relaxation and reduce physical stress.

Journaling: Writing down your thoughts helps process emotions and clear mental clutter, easing the burden on your adrenal system.

4. Support Recovery with Regular Rhythms

Your adrenal glands thrive on consistency. **Reset your natural rhythms by:**

Waking and going to bed at the same time each day, even on weekends.

Eating meals at regular intervals to maintain steady blood sugar levels.

Spending time outdoors daily, especially in the morning, to reset your circadian rhythm and encourage hormonal balance.

5. Detoxify Your Body and Environment

Toxins in your environment can further stress your adrenal glands. **To detoxify:**

Choose natural, chemical-free cleaning and personal care products.

Include detoxifying foods like cruciferous vegetables, garlic, and fresh herbs in your diet.

Sweat regularly through exercise or saunas to aid in toxin elimination.

6. Incorporate Gentle, Hormone-Balancing Exercise

While high-intensity workouts can strain your adrenal glands, gentle movement helps restore balance. **Opt for:**

Walking, swimming, or tai chi.

Strength training sessions that are moderate in intensity.

Restorative yoga to calm your nervous system.

7. Supplement Wisely

Sometimes, your body needs extra support to replenish depleted reserves. Consider these supplements under the **guidance of a healthcare professional:**

Vitamin C: A key nutrient for adrenal health.

B Vitamins: Especially B5 and B6, which support adrenal hormone production.

Magnesium: Reduces stress and promotes relaxation.

Adaptogens: As mentioned earlier, these herbs are a cornerstone of natural adrenal support.

Transforming Your Life Through Adrenal Recovery

Replenishing adrenal reserves is not just about reducing stress—it's about creating a sustainable lifestyle that supports your body's natural rhythms. As you implement these changes, you'll notice shifts in your energy, mood, and overall well-being. Your hormones will begin to rebalance, your metabolism will stabilize, and you'll feel more connected to your body.

This unique 4-week blueprint in The Hormone Reset Plan offers a step-by-step guide to help you reclaim your energy, restore balance, and transform your life naturally. By focusing on nourishing your body, calming your mind, and resetting your rhythms, you can lay the foundation for long-lasting health and vitality.

7.3 Supplements for Energy and Balance

In today's fast-paced world, fatigue and hormonal imbalances are common challenges. Often, these issues are linked to stress, poor nutrition, or lifestyle factors that disrupt the body's natural rhythms. The good news is that supplements can play a powerful role in restoring energy and balance. When combined with the strategies outlined in The Hormone Reset Plan, supplements provide essential support for your thyroid, adrenals, mood, and metabolism.

Below, we'll explore some of the most effective supplements to help you revitalize your body naturally.

Supporting Thyroid Function

Your thyroid plays a central role in regulating metabolism and energy levels. If it's underperforming, you may feel sluggish, cold, or gain weight easily. **These supplements can help:**

1. Iodine

Why: Essential for the production of thyroid hormones, iodine supports the thyroid gland's function.

Sources: Look for iodine from kelp or other sea-based supplements.

2. Selenium

Why: Selenium protects the thyroid from oxidative damage and aids in converting T4 (inactive hormone) to T3 (active hormone).

Sources: Brazil nut-derived selenium or capsule form.

3. Zinc and Copper

Why: These trace minerals work together to support thyroid hormone production and overall energy metabolism.

Note: Use a balanced formula to prevent one mineral from dominating.

Recharging Your Adrenals

Your adrenal glands manage stress by producing hormones like cortisol and adrenaline. Chronic stress can leave them depleted, leading to exhaustion and imbalanced hormones. **To nurture adrenal health:**

1. Vitamin C

Why: The adrenal glands store more vitamin C than any other organ, and it's vital for stress hormone production.

Sources: Look for liposomal vitamin C for better absorption.

2. Adaptogenic Herbs (Ashwagandha and Rhodiola)

Why: These herbs help your body adapt to stress, improving resilience and reducing cortisol levels.

Usage: Choose high-quality extracts standardized for active compounds.

3. Magnesium Glycinate

Why: Magnesium calms the nervous system and supports adrenal recovery.

Usage: Take at night to promote restful sleep.

Boosting Mood and Mental Clarity

Hormonal imbalances can wreak havoc on your mood, leaving you feeling anxious, irritable, or depressed. The right supplements can stabilize neurotransmitters and enhance emotional well-being.

1. Omega-3 Fatty Acids

Why: Omega-3s from fish oil reduce inflammation and support brain health, which is critical for hormone balance.

Sources: Choose a high-purity, third-party-tested fish oil.

2. B Vitamins (B6, B9, B12)

Why: These vitamins support the production of serotonin and dopamine, the "feel-good" chemicals in the brain.

Usage: Opt for a methylated B-complex for better absorption.

3. Probiotics

Why: A healthy gut influences mood by promoting the production of serotonin.

Sources: Look for multi-strain probiotics with billions of active cultures.

Enhancing Metabolism

A sluggish metabolism can make weight management and energy regulation difficult. **These supplements can provide the boost you need:**

1. L-Carnitine

Why: This amino acid helps transport fat into cells to be burned for energy, supporting weight loss and endurance.

Usage: Take before physical activity for optimal results.

2. Chromium Picolinate

Why: Chromium stabilizes blood sugar levels, reducing energy crashes and cravings.

Sources: Often combined with other metabolism-boosting nutrients.

3. Coenzyme Q10 (CoQ10)

Why: A powerful antioxidant that fuels energy production in every cell.

Usage: Look for ubiquinol, the active form of CoQ10, for better absorption.

A Holistic Approach

Supplements are a critical piece of the puzzle, but they work best when paired with lifestyle changes. Prioritize nutrient-dense meals, restorative sleep, regular movement, and mindfulness practices to maximize your results.

Remember, consistency is key. Over the next four weeks, let these supplements complement your commitment to The Hormone Reset Plan. By the end of the program, you'll feel more energetic, balanced, and ready to reclaim your life.

Chapter 8

Building Restful Sleep and Recovery

8.1 The Sleep-Hormone Connection

Sleep is more than just a nightly pause; it's the cornerstone of your hormonal health. When sleep is disrupted, your body's intricate hormonal system can spiral into imbalance, leading to issues like weight gain, fatigue, mood swings, and even chronic diseases. Understanding the link between sleep and hormones is essential for reclaiming your health, energy, and vitality.

How Sleep Impacts Your Hormones

During sleep, your body doesn't just rest—it regenerates, repairs, and recalibrates. Several hormones are directly influenced by the quality and quantity of your sleep:

1. Cortisol: The Stress Hormone

Cortisol naturally peaks in the morning, helping you wake up alert and energized. Poor sleep disrupts this rhythm, causing cortisol levels to spike at night when they should be low. This leads to difficulty falling or staying asleep and a vicious cycle of stress and exhaustion.

2. Melatonin: The Sleep Hormone

Melatonin is your body's natural signal for sleep, rising as darkness falls and decreasing as daylight approaches. Exposure to artificial light—particularly from screens—can suppress melatonin production, delaying sleep and disrupting its restorative benefits.

3. Growth Hormone: For Repair and Renewal

Deep sleep is when growth hormone is at its peak. This hormone is crucial for cellular repair, muscle growth, and maintaining a youthful metabolism. Without enough deep sleep, your body struggles to heal and rejuvenate, leaving you feeling drained.

4. Insulin: The Blood Sugar Regulator

Sleep deprivation can make your cells less responsive to insulin, increasing your risk of insulin resistance and weight gain. Balanced sleep helps your body maintain stable blood sugar levels and supports a healthy metabolism.

5. Leptin and Ghrelin: Appetite Controllers

These hormones regulate hunger and fullness. Sleep deprivation lowers leptin (the hormone that signals fullness) and increases ghrelin (the hormone that signals hunger). This imbalance often leads to overeating, especially cravings for sugary and high-calorie foods.

The Sleep-Hormone Cycle: A Two-Way Street

Just as sleep influences hormones, hormones also affect sleep. Imbalances in thyroid hormones, cortisol, or sex hormones like estrogen and progesterone can disrupt sleep patterns. For instance, elevated cortisol levels from chronic stress can keep you awake, while low progesterone in women, especially during menopause, can lead to insomnia.

Practical Steps to Improve Sleep and Balance Hormones

1. Prioritize a Consistent Sleep Schedule
Go to bed and wake up at the same time every day, even on weekends. This helps regulate your body's internal clock and supports consistent hormone production.

2. Create a Sleep-Friendly Environment
Keep your bedroom cool, dark, and quiet. Invest in blackout curtains and eliminate electronic devices that emit blue light, which interferes with melatonin production.

3. Limit Caffeine and Alcohol
Both substances can disrupt sleep and alter hormone levels. Avoid caffeine after midday and limit alcohol, especially in the evening.

4. Practice Relaxation Techniques

Engage in activities that lower cortisol, such as meditation, deep breathing, or gentle yoga, particularly before bedtime. These practices help calm your nervous system and prepare your body for restful sleep.

5. Support Your Sleep with Nutrition

Include foods rich in tryptophan (like turkey, nuts, and seeds), magnesium (like leafy greens and almonds), and B vitamins to support melatonin and serotonin production.

6. Stay Active, but Time It Right

Regular exercise supports hormone balance, but intense workouts late in the evening can elevate cortisol and disrupt sleep. Aim for morning or early afternoon activity.

By understanding and addressing the sleep-hormone connection, you can reset your body's natural rhythms, reclaim your energy, and transform your life. Sleep is not a luxury—it's a non-negotiable for hormonal health and overall well-being.

8.2 Creating a Bedtime Routine That Heals

In today's fast-paced world, quality sleep is often overlooked, yet it plays a critical role in hormonal balance, overall health, and emotional well-being. A consistent and mindful bedtime routine can be transformative, offering not just rest but also healing. This section delves into how you can create a bedtime routine that works for you, supports your body's natural rhythms, and helps reset your hormones.

Why a Bedtime Routine Matters

Your body thrives on rhythm. The circadian rhythm, often referred to as your internal clock, governs processes like hormone production, metabolism, and energy levels. When this rhythm is disrupted by irregular sleep patterns, late-night screen time, or chronic stress, your hormonal balance suffers. Key hormones like melatonin, cortisol, and growth hormone are particularly sensitive to your sleep-wake cycle.

By establishing a consistent bedtime routine, you signal to your body that it's time to unwind, rest, and repair. This promotes deep, restorative sleep, which is essential for hormone reset and overall vitality.

Steps to Create a Healing Bedtime Routine

1. Set a Consistent Sleep Schedule
Aim to go to bed and wake up at the same time every day—even on weekends. This consistency strengthens your circadian rhythm, ensuring that hormone production aligns with your body's needs.

2. Create a Sleep-Inducing Environment
Transform your bedroom into a sanctuary for rest. Keep it dark, quiet, and cool, as these conditions optimize melatonin production. Consider blackout curtains, a white noise machine, or a fan to enhance your sleep environment.

3. Limit Exposure to Screens

The blue light emitted by phones, tablets, and computers interferes with melatonin release, delaying sleep. Power down devices at least one hour before bedtime and replace screen time with calming activities like reading, journaling, or meditating.

4. Wind Down with Relaxation Techniques
Incorporate relaxation practices to calm your mind and body. **These could include:**

Gentle stretching or yoga: Loosens tension and prepares your body for rest.

Deep breathing or meditation: Slows your heart rate and reduces cortisol levels.

Warm bath or shower: The drop in body temperature after bathing signals your body it's time for sleep.

5. Embrace Sleep-Supportive Nutrition
Steer clear of large meals, stimulants like caffeine, and alcoholic drinks in the hours

leading up to bedtime. Instead, opt for a small snack that supports sleep, such as a banana with almond butter or a warm cup of chamomile tea. Foods rich in magnesium and tryptophan help your body relax and promote restful sleep.

6. Reflect and Express Gratitude
End your day on a positive note by reflecting on the day's achievements and expressing gratitude. Journaling a few things you're thankful for shifts your focus away from stress and creates a sense of peace before bed.

The Healing Power of Restful Sleep

When you establish and stick to a bedtime routine, you allow your body to enter its natural healing state. During deep sleep, your body repairs tissues, strengthens the immune system, and regulates hormones like leptin and ghrelin, which influence appetite and metabolism. Sleep also plays a crucial role in emotional regulation, helping to reduce anxiety and improve mood.

A healing bedtime routine is not about perfection—it's about consistency. Start small, choose one or two steps to implement, and build from there. Over time, these simple changes will create a ripple effect, enhancing not only your sleep quality but also your overall health, energy, and well-being.

By nurturing your body with restful sleep, you're giving yourself one of the most powerful tools for resetting your hormones and reclaiming your energy. Healing begins when you prioritize rest—because a balanced life starts with a balanced bedtime.

Week 4: Sustain and Thrive

Chapter 9

Maintaining Hormonal Balance Long-Term

9.1 Reinforcing Healthy Habits

As you enter the fourth week of The Hormone Reset Plan, you're standing at a powerful crossroads. By now, you've planted the seeds of transformation—adjusting your diet, improving sleep, managing stress, and incorporating exercise. This week is about solidifying those changes into lifelong habits that not only balance your hormones but also rebuild trust in your body's ability to heal itself.

Here's how to make the most of this pivotal week:

Celebrate Your Progress

Take a moment to reflect on how far you've come. Recognizing your achievements, no matter how small, builds momentum and reinforces positive change. Did your energy improve? Is your mood more stable? Are you sleeping better? Celebrate these wins. Gratitude for progress, rather than perfection, fosters resilience.

Action Tip:
Write down three positive changes you've experienced since starting this journey. Let this list remind you of why you began and how much you've already accomplished.

Fine-Tune Your Routine
Habits are strongest when they fit seamlessly into your daily life. By week four, you'll notice which practices come naturally and which ones need tweaking. Adjust your plan to match your unique needs while staying true to the core principles.

Diet: Stick to whole, unprocessed foods that nourish your hormones. If you've experimented with reducing sugar, caffeine, or processed foods, evaluate how these changes feel.

Exercise: Consistency is key. Choose activities you enjoy to ensure long-term adherence, whether it's yoga, walking, or strength training.

Sleep: Protect your bedtime routine. Deep, restorative sleep is essential for hormonal balance.

Action Tip:
Revisit your daily schedule and identify any barriers. Maybe mornings work better for workouts, or prepping meals on Sundays saves weekday stress. Small adjustments can yield big results.

Anchor New Habits with a "Why"

Understanding why you're making these changes strengthens your commitment. For example, if your goal is to improve energy, remind yourself of the joy you'll feel being fully present with loved ones. Connecting habits to deeper values turns them into lifestyle choices rather than fleeting resolutions.

Action Tip:
Write a short affirmation like, "I prioritize my health so I can show up for the people and activities I love." Place it somewhere visible—your mirror, journal, or phone lock screen.

Guard Against Setbacks

Progress often invites temptation. You may feel the urge to return to old habits, especially if life gets stressful. This week, focus on building strategies to stay on track when challenges arise.

Mindset: A slip is not a failure; it's a learning opportunity. Reflect on what triggered the setback and plan to handle it differently next time.

Environment: Remove triggers that lead to unhealthy habits. Stock your home with nutrient-dense foods and create spaces for relaxation.

Support: Lean on your support system. Share your goals with friends, family, or a health coach who can encourage and motivate you.

Action Tip:
Plan for obstacles. For example, if you're attending a social event, decide in advance how you'll navigate food choices. This empowers you to stay consistent without feeling deprived.

The Power of Consistency

Consistency is the cornerstone of habit reinforcement. Remember, small daily actions compound over time. A morning walk, a calming breath before meals, or choosing water over soda may seem minor, but these choices lay the foundation for lasting health.

Action Tip:

Track your habits using a simple checklist or app. Seeing your progress visually can boost your motivation and help you stay accountable.

Prepare for What's Next

As this four-week reset concludes, think of it as the beginning of a lifelong commitment to self-care. Your hormones thrive on stability, so staying consistent is key. Use this week to establish a sustainable rhythm that keeps your energy high, your mood balanced, and your metabolism humming.

You've taken remarkable steps to reclaim your health and balance your hormones naturally. The journey doesn't end here—it evolves with you. By reinforcing the healthy habits you've cultivated, you're not just resetting your body; you're rewriting your story. Trust in the process, celebrate your resilience, and honor the progress you've made.

This final week is your invitation to solidify a healthier, more energized version of yourself. Remember, this plan is not a sprint; it's a marathon of love and care for your body. Stay the course, and let your transformation inspire others around you.

9.2 Adapting to Seasonal and Life Changes

Adapting to seasonal and life changes is the final cornerstone in The Hormone Reset Plan. By the fourth week, you've already built a foundation for balancing your hormones, reclaiming energy, and improving overall well-being. Now, it's time to anchor these habits into your daily life, creating resilience against the inevitable shifts that come with changing seasons and life transitions.

Understanding Seasonal and Life Shifts

Our bodies are deeply connected to the rhythms of nature. The change of seasons can influence everything from sleep patterns and energy levels to mood and metabolism. Similarly, life transitions—whether it's a new job, pregnancy, menopause, or retirement—can challenge our hormonal balance and overall health.

During this week, the goal is to cultivate flexibility and resilience, ensuring your body and mind are equipped to handle these changes without feeling depleted.

1. Adjusting Your Diet to Seasonal Needs

Nature provides foods that align with our body's needs throughout the year.

Spring: Focus on detoxifying greens like spinach, arugula, and dandelion. These foods help cleanse the liver and reset your metabolism.

Summer: Stay hydrated and incorporate cooling foods like cucumbers, watermelon, and leafy salads.

Fall: Transition to grounding foods such as root vegetables, squashes, and warm soups, which support the digestive system.

Winter: Embrace nutrient-dense, warming meals like stews, whole grains, and healthy fats (avocados, nuts, and seeds) to keep your energy steady.

Tip: Maintain hormonal balance by incorporating seasonal superfoods rich in antioxidants, vitamins, and minerals.

2. Prioritizing Rest and Recovery

Seasonal changes and life transitions can disrupt your sleep and stress levels, affecting the adrenals and thyroid. In Week 4, take your self-care up a notch:

Optimize sleep: Shorter days in winter call for earlier bedtimes. Adjust your routine to align with natural daylight cycles.

Manage stress: Use deep breathing, mindfulness, or yoga to navigate life's unpredictability without overwhelming your adrenals.

Key Practice: Honor your body's natural rhythms. A slower pace during winter or stressful transitions allows time for renewal and healing.

3. Tailoring Movement to Seasonal Energy Levels

Physical activity is essential for hormonal balance, but your approach should adapt to the season or life stage:

Spring/Summer: Engage in energizing activities like running, swimming, or outdoor sports.

Fall/Winter: Transition to gentle exercises such as walking, Pilates, or restorative yoga to conserve energy.

During Transitions: Listen to your body. If you're recovering from stress or a major life event, prioritize rest over high-intensity workouts.

4. Boosting Mood Through Light Exposure and Connection

Seasonal shifts, especially in darker months, can impact mood and hormonal health, particularly serotonin and melatonin production. **Combat these challenges with:**

Natural light: Spend at least 15–30 minutes outdoors daily, even in winter, to regulate circadian rhythms.

Social support: Life changes can feel isolating. Stay connected with supportive friends or join communities that align with your goals.

Vitamin D: Ensure adequate levels through supplementation or sun exposure to support thyroid and bone health.

5. Staying Consistent with Your Reset Plan

Life will always bring unexpected challenges. What matters most is consistency, not perfection. Small, steady habits built over the past three weeks will serve as your foundation, even during tougher times.

Meal prep in advance: When life gets busy, having healthy options ready can keep you on track.

Set realistic goals: During transitions, focus on maintaining the basics—balanced meals, hydration, and rest.

Reflect and adapt: Use journaling to track your progress, note what works, and make adjustments as needed.

A Lifelong Blueprint for Resilience

Adapting to seasonal and life changes is not about drastic overhauls. It's about understanding your body's needs and making gentle adjustments that keep you balanced and energized.

By the end of this fourth week, you'll have the tools to face every season—and every life stage—with confidence and grace. You've reset your hormones, reclaimed your energy, and developed a lifestyle that supports long-term health. This is your new foundation, and it's built to last.

This week marks the culmination of your journey, but it's also a new beginning. The habits you've formed are more than a plan—they're a way of life. You're now equipped to thrive, no matter what changes come your way.

9.3 Setting Up a Weekly Self-Care Routine

Congratulations on making it to Week 4 of your journey toward hormonal balance and renewed vitality. By this stage, you've laid a strong foundation for your health and well-being. The final week is about refining the strategies you've practiced and transforming them into a consistent, sustainable self-care routine that supports your body long-term.

Why a Weekly Self-Care Routine Matters

Hormonal health is not a one-time fix but a dynamic, ongoing process. Life's stressors, nutritional gaps, and even small shifts in sleep patterns can throw your body out of balance. A thoughtfully designed weekly self-care routine provides structure, reduces overwhelm, and allows your body to stay resilient, even during challenging times.

This week, we focus on integrating the strategies you've learned so they become second nature. A weekly rhythm reduces decision fatigue and ensures that you consistently prioritize activities that nourish your thyroid, adrenals, metabolism, and overall well-being.

Key Components of Your Weekly Self-Care Plan

Your routine doesn't need to be rigid or complicated; it simply needs to address the core areas of hormonal health: sleep, nutrition, movement, stress management, and connection. **Below is a guide to crafting a comprehensive yet flexible weekly plan:**

1. Prioritize Quality Sleep

Why: Sleep is your hormonal reset button. It allows your body to repair, detoxify, and regulate cortisol and melatonin levels.

What to Do:

Commit to 7–9 hours of sleep each night.

Establish a "wind-down" ritual 30–60 minutes before bed, such as turning off screens, dimming the lights, or sipping calming herbal tea.

Choose one night per week to go to bed an hour earlier than usual for additional recovery.

2. Plan Your Meals and Snacks

Why: Balanced nutrition stabilizes blood sugar, reduces inflammation, and fuels your metabolism.

What to Do:

Spend 1–2 hours on a specific day (e.g., Sunday or Monday) to prep meals for the week. Focus on nutrient-dense, hormone-friendly foods, such as lean proteins, healthy fats, and fiber-rich vegetables.

Incorporate hormone-boosting snacks into your routine, such as a handful of walnuts, an avocado smoothie, or boiled eggs with sea salt.

Use your meal-prepping time to reflect on any dietary triggers from the past week and make adjustments.

3. Schedule Time for Movement

Why: Physical activity enhances circulation, supports adrenal health, and helps regulate cortisol and insulin levels.

What to Do:

Block out at least three sessions of moderate exercise (e.g., walking, yoga, or Pilates) in your calendar.

Dedicate one day to restorative movement, such as stretching or light yoga, to help your body recover.

Consider short daily bursts of movement, such as 10 minutes of gentle stretching in the morning or evening.

4. Integrate Stress-Management Practices

Why: Chronic stress disrupts hormonal balance, leading to fatigue, mood swings, and weight gain.

What to Do:

Schedule at least 15–20 minutes of relaxation daily. Options include meditation, journaling, or deep breathing exercises.

Choose one day per week to practice a longer form of stress relief, like a nature walk, a bath infused with calming essential oils, or a creative hobby you enjoy.

Reflect on your stress triggers and develop a plan to address or reframe them.

5. Foster Social and Emotional Connection

Why: Positive relationships and emotional support play a crucial role in stabilizing cortisol and oxytocin levels.

What to Do:

Set aside time each week to connect with loved ones, whether through a shared meal, a phone call, or a simple activity like watching a movie together.

Spend time with people who uplift and inspire you, and minimize interactions that drain your energy.

Cultivate self-compassion by scheduling time to check in with yourself. Journaling or mindfulness exercises can help you tune in to your emotional needs.

Creating a Routine That Sticks

As you refine your weekly self-care routine, keep these tips in mind:

1. Keep It Realistic: Avoid overloading your schedule. A routine is effective only if it feels manageable and enjoyable.

2. Be Flexible: Life happens, and some weeks won't go as planned. Focus on progress, not perfection.

3. Celebrate Small Wins: Acknowledge the positive changes you've made and how they've impacted your energy, mood, and overall health.

As you move beyond the four-week reset, remember that self-care is a journey, not a destination. Your body thrives on consistency, but it also appreciates grace. By committing to a weekly routine tailored to your needs, you'll continue to support your hormones, reclaim your energy, and transform your life.

Take time to honor your progress, no matter how small it may seem. You've done incredible work, and this routine is your key to sustaining it.

Chapter 10

Detoxifying Your Lifestyle

10.1 Transitioning to Clean Personal Care Products

Your personal care products play a surprisingly significant role in your hormonal health. Many conventional shampoos, lotions, deodorants, and cosmetics contain chemicals that can disrupt your endocrine system, throwing your hormones out of balance. Transitioning to clean personal care products is not just a trend; it's a powerful step toward supporting your body's natural balance, boosting your energy, and improving your overall well-being.

The Problem with Conventional Products

Every day, we are exposed to ingredients like parabens, phthalates, synthetic fragrances, and sulfates in our personal care routines. These substances are often classified as endocrine disruptors, meaning they can mimic or interfere with hormones like estrogen, testosterone, and thyroid hormones. Over time, this exposure can contribute to issues like fatigue, weight gain, mood swings, and even chronic conditions.

Your skin, the largest organ in your body, absorbs a significant portion of what you apply to it. This means that your lotion or shampoo may do more than moisturize or cleanse—it can also deliver harmful chemicals into your bloodstream. Transitioning to cleaner, safer alternatives helps reduce this toxic load, giving your body a chance to rebalance itself naturally.

Why Transitioning Matters for Hormone Health

1. Restores Balance
Switching to non-toxic products reduces the chemical interference in your hormone production and regulation. This can lead to clearer skin, better sleep, more stable moods, and enhanced energy levels.

2. Supports Detoxification
Clean products reduce the burden on your liver, which plays a crucial role in metabolizing and detoxifying hormones. A lower toxic load means your liver can focus on maintaining hormonal harmony.

3. Promotes Longevity
Reducing exposure to harmful chemicals decreases the risk of long-term health issues such as reproductive disorders, autoimmune diseases, and certain cancers.

How to Transition Effectively

1. Start Small, Think Big
You don't have to replace all your products at once. Begin with the items you use daily and on large areas of your body, such as body wash, lotion, and deodorant. Gradually work your way through your entire routine.

2. Read Labels Carefully

When shopping for clean products, look for certifications like USDA Organic, EWG Verified, or COSMOS Natural. Avoid products with synthetic fragrances, parabens, sulfates, and phthalates. If you're unsure about an ingredient, research it or consult apps like Think Dirty or EWG's Skin Deep Database.

3. Focus on Simplified Formulas
Choose products with fewer ingredients, especially ones you recognize, like coconut oil, shea butter, or essential oils. Simpler formulations are often gentler and safer.

4. DIY When Possible
Homemade personal care products allow you to control what goes into them. For example, you can create a simple deodorant using baking soda, coconut oil, and essential oils or a nourishing face mask with honey and turmeric.

5. Be Patient with Your Body
When transitioning, your body may go through an adjustment period. For example, switching to

a natural deodorant may result in increased sweating initially as your body detoxifies. Stick with it—these temporary changes often lead to lasting improvements.

The Hormone-Reset Friendly Routine

Incorporating clean personal care products is a natural extension of The Hormone Reset Plan. By eliminating unnecessary toxins, you allow your body to heal, restore, and thrive. Each small change you make is a step closer to reclaiming your energy and transforming your life.

Your personal care routine should nourish you, not burden you. As you transition, remember: this isn't about perfection but progress. With every product you switch to a cleaner alternative, you empower your body to find its balance naturally.

10.2 DIY Natural Cleaning Solutions

Maintaining a clean home is essential to your health, especially when trying to balance your hormones. Traditional cleaning products often contain harsh chemicals that disrupt your endocrine system, aggravating hormonal imbalances. By switching to natural, DIY cleaning solutions, you can create a safer environment that supports your hormone reset journey.

Here are some simple, effective recipes for natural cleaning products, complete with clear instructions and ingredients.

1. All-Purpose Cleaning Spray

This versatile cleaner can be used on countertops, tables, and most surfaces.

Ingredients:

- 2 cups distilled water

- 1 cup white vinegar

- 1 tablespoon baking soda

- 10 drops lemon essential oil (optional for scent and antibacterial properties)

- 10 drops tea tree essential oil (antimicrobial and antifungal properties)

Instructions:

1. In a spray bottle, combine the distilled water and white vinegar.

2. Slowly add the baking soda to prevent fizzing overflow.

3. Add the essential oils for scent and extra cleaning power.

4. Shake well before each use. Spray onto surfaces and wipe with a clean cloth.

2. Natural Glass Cleaner

Get streak-free windows and mirrors with this eco-friendly cleaner.

Ingredients:

- 2 cups distilled water

- 1/4 cup white vinegar

- 1/4 cup rubbing alcohol (70% concentration)

- 1 tablespoon cornstarch (helps reduce streaks)

- 5 drops lavender essential oil (optional for scent)

Instructions:

1. Mix all ingredients in a spray bottle.

2. Shake well to ensure the cornstarch dissolves completely.

3. Spray onto glass surfaces and wipe with a microfiber cloth or newspaper for a streak-free shine.

3. Homemade Floor Cleaner

This solution works well on tile, laminate, or hardwood floors.

Ingredients:

- 1 gallon warm water

- 1/2 cup white vinegar

- 1/4 cup liquid castile soap

- 10 drops eucalyptus essential oil (antimicrobial and refreshing scent)

Instructions:

1. In a large bucket, mix the warm water, vinegar, and castile soap.

2. Add the essential oil for a fresh scent.

3. Dip a mop into the mixture, wring out excess liquid, and clean the floors as usual.

4. Natural Toilet Bowl Cleaner

Keep your bathroom fresh and free from harsh chemicals.

Ingredients:

- 1/2 cup baking soda

- 1/4 cup white vinegar

- 10 drops tea tree essential oil (antibacterial and antifungal properties)

Instructions:

1. Sprinkle the baking soda inside the toilet bowl.

2. Pour the vinegar over the baking soda to create a fizzing reaction.

3. Add tea tree essential oil for additional cleaning power.

4. Scrub the bowl with a toilet brush, then flush.

5. DIY Laundry Detergent

Reduce exposure to synthetic fragrances and detergents with this natural alternative.

Ingredients:

- 1 bar castile soap, grated

- 1 cup washing soda (sodium carbonate)

- 1 cup borax (optional, for whitening and deodorizing)

- 10 drops lemon or lavender essential oil (optional)

Instructions:

1. In a large bowl, mix the grated soap, washing soda, and borax.

2. Add the essential oil for a pleasant scent.

3. Store the mixture in an airtight container. Use 2 tablespoons per load of laundry.

Benefits of DIY Natural Cleaning Solutions

1. Non-Toxic Environment: Protects your body from hormone-disrupting chemicals.

2. Cost-Effective: Saves money compared to store-bought alternatives.

3. Eco-Friendly: Reduces your carbon footprint with biodegradable ingredients.

4. Customizable: Adjust scents and strengths to your preference.

Incorporating these natural cleaning solutions into your routine supports the hormone reset plan by minimizing your exposure to harmful chemicals. A clean home, free from toxins, creates a supportive foundation for balancing your body, reclaiming your energy, and transforming your life.

10.3 Reducing Environmental Stressors

In today's world, the environment around us plays a pivotal role in shaping our health and hormonal balance. Many of the products, habits, and surroundings we interact with daily contain hidden stressors that can disrupt our body's natural harmony. Addressing these environmental factors is a cornerstone of The Hormone Reset Plan, helping you balance your body, reclaim your energy, and transform your life.

The Impact of Environmental Stressors on Hormones

Your hormones act as messengers that regulate critical functions, including metabolism, mood, energy levels, and sleep. Unfortunately, environmental stressors such as toxins, pollutants, and even electromagnetic radiation can interfere with these processes. Prolonged exposure to these factors may lead to hormonal imbalances, contributing to symptoms like fatigue, weight gain, mood swings, and poor sleep.

Reducing environmental stressors helps your body recover, reset, and maintain optimal hormone function. It's about creating a cleaner, safer space that supports healing and vitality.

Key Environmental Stressors to Address

1. Toxins in Household Products
Many cleaning supplies, personal care products, and plastics contain harmful chemicals, such as

endocrine disruptors, which mimic or interfere with hormone function. **Common culprits include:**

Phthalates: Found in fragranced products like air fresheners and shampoos.

BPA: Found in plastics and food packaging.

Parabens: Found in cosmetics and skincare products.

What to do:

Switch to natural, fragrance-free cleaning supplies.

Choose glass or stainless steel containers for food storage.

Opt for skincare products with simple, organic ingredients.

2. Air Quality and Pollutants

Indoor air pollution can be a hidden stressor, with allergens, mold, and volatile organic compounds (VOCs) contributing to inflammation and stress on the body.

What to do:

Use a HEPA air filter to improve air quality.

Open windows regularly to ventilate your home.

Avoid using synthetic air fresheners or candles.

3. Water Contaminants
Tap water can contain traces of heavy metals, pesticides, and hormone-disrupting chemicals.

What to do:

Invest in a high-quality water filtration system.

Use stainless steel or glass water bottles to avoid leaching plastics.

4. Electromagnetic Radiation (EMFs)
Constant exposure to electronic devices, Wi-Fi, and cell towers can contribute to stress and poor sleep, both of which affect hormone balance.

What to do:

Turn off Wi-Fi at night.

Use wired connections where possible.

Keep devices away from your body, especially while sleeping.

5. Clutter and Noise Pollution
A cluttered, chaotic environment can lead to chronic low-level stress, which disrupts cortisol regulation. Noise pollution, like loud traffic or constant electronic sounds, can also elevate stress hormones.

What to do:

Declutter your living and working spaces regularly.

Create a quiet, restful area for relaxation and meditation.

Use noise-canceling devices or white noise machines to block out disruptive sounds.

Steps to Create a Hormone-Friendly Environment

1. Conduct an Environmental Audit
Take a close look at your home, workspace, and daily habits. Identify potential stressors like toxic products, poor air quality, or excessive screen time.

2. Prioritize Clean Eating and Storage
Choose organic, minimally processed foods to reduce exposure to pesticides and additives. Store food in non-toxic containers like glass or stainless steel.

3. Embrace Natural Light and Nature

Spending time outdoors and getting natural sunlight helps regulate your circadian rhythm and supports melatonin production, essential for restful sleep. Incorporating plants indoors can also improve air quality and promote a sense of calm.

4. Commit to a Daily Detox

Support your body's natural detoxification processes through hydration, exercise, and antioxidant-rich foods. Sweating during physical activity can help flush out toxins, while leafy greens and cruciferous vegetables support liver function.

The Long-Term Benefits

By addressing environmental stressors, you'll notice improvements in your energy, mood, and overall health. Hormonal balance is not just about managing symptoms—it's about creating a lifestyle that allows your body to thrive.

With small, consistent changes, you can transform your environment into a sanctuary for healing and vitality. This process is a powerful step in The Hormone Reset Plan, helping you take control of your health and reclaim the vibrant life you deserve.

www.ingramcontent.com/pod-product-compliance
Lightning Source LLC
Chambersburg PA
CBHW071022240526
45469CB00006BD/2045